STROKE

**Questions
you
have
. . . Answers
you
need**

Other Books From The People's Medical Society

Take This Book to the Hospital With You

How to Evaluate and Select a Nursing Home

Medicine on Trial

Medicare Made Easy

Your Medical Rights

Getting the Most for Your Medical Dollar

Take This Book to the Gynecologist With You

Take This Book to the Obstetrician With You

Blood Pressure: Questions You Have . . . Answers You Need

Your Heart: Questions You Have . . . Answers You Need

The Consumer's Guide to Medical Lingo

150 Ways to Be a Savvy Medical Consumer

Take This Book to the Pediatrician With You

100 Ways to Live to 100

Dial 800 for Health

Your Complete Medical Record

Arthritis: Questions You Have . . . Answers You Need

Diabetes: Questions You Have . . . Answers You Need

Prostate: Questions You Have . . . Answers You Need

Vitamins and Minerals: Questions You Have . . . Answers You Need

Good Operations—Bad Operations

The Complete Book of Relaxation Techniques

Test Yourself for Maximum Health

Misdiagnosis: Woman As a Disease

Yoga Made Easy

Massage Made Easy

Hearing Loss: Questions You Have . . . Answers You Need

Asthma: Questions You Have . . . Answers You Need

Depression: Questions You Have . . . Answers You Need

Back Pain: Questions You Have . . . Answers You Need

STROKE

Questions
you
have
... Answers
you
need

By Jennifer Hay

≡People's Medical Society®

Allentown, Pennsylvania

The People's Medical Society is a nonprofit consumer health organization dedicated to the principles of better, more responsive and less expensive medical care. Organized in 1983, the People's Medical Society puts previously unavailable medical information into the hands of consumers so that they can make informed decisions about their own health care.

Membership in the People's Medical Society is $20 a year and includes a subscription to the *People's Medical Society Newsletter.* For information, write to the People's Medical Society, 462 Walnut Street, Allentown, PA 18102, or call 610-770-1670.

This and other People's Medical Society publications are available for quantity purchase at discount. Contact the People's Medical Society for details.

Library of Congress Cataloging-in-Publication Data
Hay, Jennifer, 1964–
    Stroke : questions you have—answers you need /
by Jennifer Hay.
      p. cm.
    Includes bibliographical references and index.
    ISBN 1-882606-22-1 (trade paper)
    1. Cerebrovascular disease—Miscellanea. I. Title.
RC388.5.H39 1995
616.8'1—dc20   95-21858
                                             CIP

1 2 3 4 5 6 7 8 9 0
First printing, July 1995

CONTENTS

INTRODUCTION

When I think of stroke, I think of quietness. For some reason, when stroke is mentioned, most people become quiet and silent. Maybe it's because the effects of a stroke can be so devastating. Maybe it's the thought of someone being paralyzed and helpless. Maybe the hush occurs because we are trying to contemplate how family and friends will handle the myriad problems that can accompany a stroke.

Most of us have a limited knowledge of strokes. Our general perception is someone paralyzed, unable to manage his daily life functions—a person closed off from a world previously enjoyed. Indeed, that can certainly be the situation, but strokes come in many forms, many of which involve no paralysis whatsoever. And stroke does not necessarily mean the end of a person's existence or independence.

In *Stroke: Questions You Have ... Answers You Need,* we present the information every person should know about strokes and their treatment. I am sure you will be surprised to learn not only of the types of strokes and their possible effects, but also of the wealth of treatments available to help the stroke victim overcome his disabilities and return to as normal a life as possible. You will also find the many ways a family can organize the home and schedule to accommodate a person who has had a stroke as he works toward regaining his previous skills.

Years ago, a stroke was either a death sentence or a guaranteed lifetime commitment to a skilled nursing facility. But not so today. Recent medical and rehabilitative treatments have improved the prospects of stroke victims, so that they can regain many, if not all, of their former skills. And the outlook for new and more effective treatments is improving all the time.

Written in an easy to follow question-and-answer format, *Stroke: Questions You Have... Answers You Need* is another in the People's Medical Society's popular series of books empowering consumers with information previously not available under one cover. I am confident that you will find the book to be a practical guide to understanding and coping with stroke.

Charles B. Inlander
President
People's Medical Society

STROKE

**Questions
you
have
...Answers
you
need**

Terms printed in boldface can be found in the glossary, beginning on page 165. Only the first mention of the word in the text will be boldfaced.

We have tried to use male and female pronouns in an egalitarian manner throughout the book. Any imbalance in usage has been in the interest of readability.

1 UNDERSTANDING STROKES

Q: I'm scared to death of **stroke**. It seems so incapacitating. Everyone I know who has had a stroke has never been the same again. Is this always the case?

A: There is no question, stroke can be devastating —in fact, it kills approximately 30 percent of its victims. And stroke's physical effects—primarily paralysis and the resulting dependence—are widely feared. In fact, the majority of people interviewed in a 1994 survey indicated that they would prefer death to severe physical disability as a consequence of stroke (*Stroke,* September 1994).

But the widely held image of a comatose or wheelchair-bound individual suddenly deprived of a normal lifestyle is only one part of a more complicated picture. It is true that stroke can be severely disabling; it can rob a person of his independence, affect his abilities to think, speak, read, write or understand spoken language, or change his behavior. In other words, stroke can and does change the life of the person it affects. But stroke's effects are not always disabling, nor are they always permanent. Some strokes produce little or no disabling effects, while others produce serious effects that improve with time. In other words, there is no standard prognosis for stroke survivors.

Q: Why is that?

A: Primarily because no two strokes are exactly alike. Essentially, a stroke is a brain injury. This injury, which results from death of or damage to brain cells, can occur in any part of the brain and can vary in size and extent of damage.

As you probably know, the brain is the nerve center of the entire body. It controls all bodily functions, dividing these management duties among its different parts. The left side of the brain, for example, controls the motor functions on the right side of the body, while the right side of the brain controls the motor functions on the left. The location of a brain injury, therefore, dictates which functions will be affected, while the extent of the injury dictates the extent of the effect.

In other words, a stroke's effects are determined in part by its location and severity. They can also be impacted by the success of early treatment or lack thereof, the development of complications, the natural healing process that follows acute stroke and the success of **rehabilitation**. So stroke's effects—which can be physical, communicative, cognitive, behavioral and emotional—vary from person to person and often change over time.

Q: I'm still confused about how the location of the brain injury relates to the effects of stroke. Could you be more specific?

A: Because the right side of the brain controls the left side of the body, damage to the right side of the brain could affect functions on the left side of the person's body—usually her arm, leg or face. The brain's right side is also responsible for spatial orientation and nonverbal communication, so a stroke on the right side of the brain could also result in a variety of other problems, including time disorientation, an altered attention span and impaired thinking skills. A stroke on the left side of the brain could affect function on the right side of the body, as well as speech, communication and thinking skills, since these functions are governed by the left side of the brain.

While left- and right-sided strokes—those that affect one side of the area of the brain known as the **cerebrum** —are the most common, stroke can also affect other areas of the brain. If it strikes the **cerebellum**—the part of the brain located at the base of the skull in the rear—reflexes, balance and coordination can be affected. And if it strikes the **brain stem**, the part of the brain that joins the spine, it can affect survival functions, such as heartbeat and breathing. Finally, some strokes affect more than one part of the brain. These strokes can affect the body and its functions in numerous ways.

Q: **I think I understand. And the extent to which these functions are affected depends on the severity of the stroke?**

A: Yes. A minor stroke will likely result in minor, perhaps reversible, effects, while a major or massive stroke—one that kills or damages a large area of brain cells—will result in severe damage.

PHYSICAL EFFECTS

Q: **Okay, so what are the possible effects of stroke?**

A: Let's start with the physical effects. As you know, stroke can be very disabling. It can result in paralysis, weakness or loss of sensation, balance and coordination problems, and problems with vision, continence and the ability to swallow.

Q: Can we take a closer look at those?

A: Certainly. Let's start with the most well-known effect, paralysis. In stroke, paralysis is usually caused by damage to one side of the brain; therefore, it usually occurs on only one side of the body. This condition, known as **hemiplegia**, can affect the leg, arm and face or a combination thereof.

Similarly, a stroke victim can experience simply **hemiparesis**, or weakness on one side of the body, or **hemianesthesia**, a loss of sensation on one side of the body. When stroke affects the brain stem or multiple parts of the brain, however, both sides of the body can be affected.

Q: What kind of balance and coordination problems can stroke cause?

A: Depending on the location of the brain injury, dizziness may be a problem. This, obviously, can affect balance. Balance may also be affected by an inability to coordinate certain muscles—a condition known as **ataxia**—on one or both sides of the body.

Q: How does stroke affect vision?

A: There are several ways: Stroke can disturb eye movements, affect perception and diminish sight in one or both eyes. The most common visual problem associated with stroke is **hemianopia**, a condition that produces defective vision or blindness in half of one or both eyes. This condition, which affects peripheral vision, cannot be corrected with glasses, because it is caused by a problem in the optic nerve.

Q: How does it affect perception?

A: Hemianopia and other visual deficits caused by stroke, along with conditions like hemiplegia and hemianesthesia, may ultimately result in a loss of awareness of the affected side. This problem, known as **neglect**, may cause a stroke survivor to forget about or ignore his weaker side. He may, for example, put only one arm through a shirt sleeve or one leg through a pant leg and believe he is fully clothed; he may eat only the food on half of his plate, or bump into furniture, doors, walls and other items he fails to see or perceive.

Q: Did you say stroke can also affect continence?

A: Yes. Some stroke victims lose control over their bladders or bowels. Conversely, others have retention problems like constipation. Fortunately, the majority of these problems, which are caused either by brain damage or bladder infections, can be overcome—either through training or the use of catheters and medications.

Q: What about swallowing problems?
Can they be overcome?

A: Difficulty in swallowing, a condition known as
dysphagia, can often be overcome with therapy.
This problem plagues many stroke survivors and can affect
their ability to eat and drink. It can also result in drooling.

COMMUNICATIVE EFFECTS

Q: How can a stroke affect a person's ability
to communicate?

A: Stroke can affect communication in a number of
ways: It can physically impair a person's ability to
speak; it can affect a person's ability to recall and use
words, grammar and syntax—her ability to use language—
and it can impair her ability to understand written or
verbal communication. These impairments, which range
from occasional speech slurring to a complete inability to
communicate, may take a variety of forms.

Q: Such as?

A: The most common impairments, in alphabetical
order, include:

• **Anomia**—a word retrieval problem: A person
may, for example, recognize an item but have difficulty
recalling its name.

• **Aphasia**—a decreased ability or an inability to
express or comprehend verbal or written language. There
are several types of aphasia:

- **Expressive aphasia** (also known as *Broca's aphasia*) is the inability to express oneself in speech or writing. A person with expressive aphasia may have things he wants to say but is unable to say them.
- **Receptive aphasia** (also known as *Wernicke's aphasia*) is the inability to comprehend written or verbal speech. A person with receptive aphasia hears what is said but cannot understand what he hears.
- **Global aphasia** is the inability to express and understand spoken or written language. In other words, it is both an expressive and receptive impairment.

There is also **jargon aphasia**, in which a person retains the ability to speak but cannot speak logically. A person with jargon aphasia may make up words, repeat one word many times or use words in ways that make no sense.

- **Dysarthria**—imperfect articulation. It occurs when the speech muscles are damaged, and its effects can range from an occasional slurred word to total unintelligibility.

- **Verbal apraxia**—the brain's impaired ability to send messages regarding speech movement to the speech muscles. People with this condition may visibly struggle to produce sounds and words. The resulting speech deficit can range from an occasional sound substitution to a complete inability to speak.

- **Paraphasia**—a partial aphasia in which a person transposes sounds or words—incorrectly substituting one word or sound for another.

It's important to remember that none of these communication problems indicates mental incompetence. In most instances, the stroke survivor knows what he wants to say; he simply cannot connect with the language center of the brain or use his speech muscles.

Q: That sounds frustrating! Are these communication problems common?

A: Yes. According to the National Institute of Neurological and Communication Diseases and Stroke, about half of all strokes result in some sort of speech difficulty. While aphasia is usually limited to people who have had left-brain strokes, dysarthria is common in both left- and right-brain strokes.

Q: Do these problems last permanently?

A: That depends. Most people who experience a communication problem naturally show some improvement, even without therapy, in the first few weeks or months. In fact, most recovery from communication deficits occurs during the first year. Some people recover completely; others retain speech and communication deficits. In many cases, speech therapy can help restore some of those lost functions.

COGNITIVE EFFECTS

Q: After learning about stroke's other effects, I'm almost afraid to ask this, but how does stroke affect the mind?

A: Stroke's cognitive effects, while not as obvious as its physical and communicative effects, can be frustrating, tragic and in some instances dangerous. Stroke can affect thinking, reasoning, memory and perception. These impairments can affect a stroke survivor's ability to perform simple tasks or make safe judgments.

Q: Exactly what effect can stroke have on thinking and reasoning?

A: Stroke can affect the ability to think clearly and the ability to reason abstractly. This can lead to short attention spans, errors in judgment, irrational behavior and impulsiveness. Sequential tasks may also become very difficult to perform. A stroke survivor, for example, might confuse the order of the steps to a certain task or forget how to perform them at all.

These difficulties can be complicated by perceptual problems, such as **agnosia**—the inability to associate an object with its use—and **apraxia**—the inability to use an object. A person with agnosia might try to brush her hair with a toothbrush or brush her teeth with a comb, while a person with apraxia may be physically capable of brushing her teeth or hair but be unable to direct her muscles to perform either action.

Q: What are some other perception problems?

A: We've already discussed neglect, which is common in stroke survivors with left-side paralysis (right-brain stroke). In addition, stroke can affect a person's ability to distinguish between foreground and background or left and right, as well as her awareness of spatial relationships. She could develop **dysmetria**, for example, which would prevent her from accurately estimating distances linked to muscle movements, such as reaching for an object. She might, for example, try to pick up a cup from a table, but underestimate the distance and grab only air; or she might try to place the cup on the table and miss, dropping it on the floor.

BEHAVIORAL AND EMOTIONAL EFFECTS

Q: Are these cognitive problems the cause of stroke's behavioral effects?

A: In part. After all, thinking does affect behavior. The shortened attention spans and impulsive behaviors common in some stroke survivors, for example, can be attributed to cognitive changes. But stroke can cause other behavioral changes—even changes in personality—that are particularly noticeable to family and friends.

Q: What kind of changes are you talking about?

A: Stroke survivors may experience a decrease in overall motivation or self-control; they may become frustrated, impatient or irritable, or behave rashly and impulsively or slowly and compulsively. They may suddenly become overtalkative or they may become socially withdrawn. They may deny their limitations or become apathetic. Or they may behave in socially inappropriate ways, demonstrating selfishness, insensitivity and tactlessness or throwing temper tantrums.

Not all stroke survivors experience all of these changes. In fact, some experience no behavioral or personality changes at all. Still, even a minor change can come as a shock if it produces behavior that differs greatly from the survivor's normal behavior. Just imagine a family's reaction when they hear their quiet, thoughtful mother babble on about nothing or see their enthusiastic father lose interest in life.

Q: Could this apathy have anything to do with depression?

A: In some cases, yes. While apathy is a common stroke effect in and of itself, it can also signal depression. And depression is quite common among stroke survivors.

Q: Why is that?

A: There are several possible explanations. In some people, particularly those whose strokes involved the front left side of their brains, depression may be directly related to the injury caused by stroke. In others, depression may be triggered by the stroke survivors' realization that their lives and lifestyles have been changed by the stroke. Perhaps they are no longer able to live independently, continue in their careers or communicate. Fortunately, however, depression can be treated, both with medications and therapy.

Q: Does stroke cause any other emotional effects?

A: Yes. Many stroke survivors cannot control their emotions, a condition known as emotional **lability**. Stroke survivors who have this problem may spontaneously laugh or cry for no obvious reason. This condition can be embarrassing for the stroke survivor and disturbing to family and friends. It does, however, usually improve somewhat over the course of months or years.

Q: I didn't realize stroke had so many wide-ranging effects. Which ones can be addressed through rehabilitation?

A: We discuss rehabilitation in Chapter 6, but first you need to know a bit more about the mechanics of stroke itself, as well as diagnosis and treatment. Let's get started.

2 BACK TO THE BASICS

Q: What exactly is stroke?

A: Essentially, stroke is an injury to the nervous system, that complex system of nerve cells (including those in the nerves, spinal cord and brain) that controls all functions of the body. This injury occurs when blood vessels fail to deliver an adequate amount of blood to the brain, which is the command center of the nervous system. And as we've said, brain injury can result in physical paralysis, weakness, visual or communication difficulties and many other neurological problems.

Q: So stroke is essentially a neurological disorder?

A: Actually, it's a cerebrovascular disorder, which means it involves both the brain and the vascular (blood vessel) system. In fact, the medical term for stroke is **cerebrovascular accident**, or **CVA**. You may also have heard it referred to as **apoplexy** or **cerebral infarction**.

Q: And this injury occurs when the brain doesn't get enough blood. Why does the brain need blood?

A: Blood supplies the body with nutrients and oxygen. And the brain, which controls most body functions, needs a lot of both. In fact, 20 percent of the heart's output of fresh blood is sent to the brain.

Q: What happens when it doesn't get enough?

A: Any disturbance in the flow of blood to the brain affects the brain's functions. Without oxygen, brain cells cannot do their job. And when the brain cells cannot function, the parts of the body they control cannot function either.

Q: Does normal function return when blood flow is restored?

A: That depends on how long the brain cells are deprived of oxygen. After a certain time without oxygen—sometimes only a matter of minutes—brain cells are injured or die. Brain cells cannot regenerate, so their death creates an area of dead tissue known as an **infarct**. This can result in permanent damage.

Q: Isn't that similar to a heart attack?

A: Yes. In fact, it's becoming increasingly common to refer to stroke as a brain attack. Both stroke and heart attack are caused by interruptions in the blood supply—interruptions that are often caused by blood clots. In both instances this interruption can create infarcts. Indeed, the medical term for heart attack is *myocardial infarction,* while the term for a stroke caused by an infarct in the brain is cerebral infarction. In addition, both conditions carry many of the same risk factors and both require immediate medical attention.

Q: How common is stroke?

A: Stroke is the third leading cause of death and the major cause of disability among American adults. According to the American Heart Association (AHA), stroke strikes an estimated 500,000 Americans each year and kills 150,000. And while more people are surviving strokes now than ever before (the death rate declined more than 50 percent between 1960 and 1990), the majority of long-term survivors still experience major changes in their lifestyles. The AHA estimates that 15 percent require institutional care; one-third depend on someone else for help in bathing, dressing, using the bathroom and other **activities of daily living**; and more than half report a decrease in their social life.

Q: I know we touched on this before, but are the effects of stroke always permanent?

A: They can be. Their permanence depends on the location and severity of the stroke, as well the stroke victim's response to rehabilitation. As the victim recovers, some problems may resolve themselves. Others may be resolved through rehabilitation and retraining. After all, it's the brain cells that are damaged, not the affected body parts. And while dead brain cells cannot regenerate, other brain cells may be trained to assume their roles.

Q: So it's possible to recover from a stroke?

A: It is. Stroke is not an automatic sentence to a life of disability. Some people emerge from a stroke unscathed, and many people have gone on to lead normal, even outstanding, lives after suffering a stroke. Louis Pasteur, for example, developed the principles of vaccination 24 years after his stroke. Composer George Frideric Handel wrote the *Messiah* four years after his stroke, and British Prime Minister Winston Churchill, poet Walt Whitman, dancer Agnes DeMille and actress Patricia Neal all continued highly visible, successful careers after having strokes. That's not to say, however, that stroke cannot be disabling. It can be, as the statistics show. In fact, there are more than 2.5 million disabled stroke survivors in the United States.

Q: All because the brain didn't get enough blood! What causes this lack of blood flow?

A: That depends on the type of stroke. In **ischemic stroke**, a blockage in a blood vessel is usually responsible; in **hemorrhagic stroke**, it is the rupture of a blood vessel.

Q: Tell me more about ischemic stroke. What could possibly block a blood vessel?

A: Blood clots are the major culprits, although other foreign material in the bloodstream can also block vessels. Low blood flow caused by a narrowing of the arteries or a heart problem can produce similar results. Both low blood flow (**hypoperfusion**) and actual blockages (**occlusions**) cause **ischemia**, an inadequate supply of blood to the brain that can result in ischemic stroke.

Q: What exactly is a blood clot?

A: A blood clot is a semisolid mass that results from the clotting process of the blood. It is composed primarily of red and white blood cells and platelets held together by a protein.

Q: Where do clots usually occur?

A: A clot, or **thrombus**, often develops in arteries that have been narrowed by a buildup of fatty deposits on the inner layers of artery walls, a condition known as **atherosclerosis**. The clot, coupled with the narrowed arteries, combines to block blood from flowing. In addition, the fatty deposits themselves can break off and block blood flow.

Q: Where do these blockages originate?

A: In **cerebral thrombosis**, the most common type of stroke, the blockage originates in an artery that supplies blood to the brain. In **cerebral embolism**, a clot or other foreign material originating elsewhere in the body is carried through the bloodstream and lodges in an artery leading to the brain. This traveling material, known as an **embolus**, often forms in the heart.

Q: You said cerebral thrombosis is the most common type of stroke. How common is it?

A: Estimates vary. According to the AHA, cerebral thrombosis accounts for between 56 and 75 percent of all strokes. Between 5 and 14 percent are caused by cerebral embolism, and the rest are caused by hemorrhages.

Q: What causes a hemorrhagic stroke?

A: Hemorrhage, or bleeding, can be caused by a head injury, the rupture of an **aneurysm** (a bulge in the wall of a blood vessel) or the leakage or rupture of a congenitally weak or malformed blood vessel.

Q: Are these actually different types of hemorrhagic stroke?

A: No. Hemorrhagic stroke type is determined by location. In **cerebral hemorrhage**, the ruptured or leaking artery is actually located in the brain tissue. In **subarachnoid hemorrhage**, the bleeding is on the surface of brain between brain and skull.

Q: Which type is more common?

A: Cerebral hemorrhage accounts for about 10 percent of all strokes, while subarachnoid hemorrhage accounts for about 7 percent, according to the AHA.

Q: Which is more serious, a hemorrhagic stroke or an ischemic stroke?

A: Both types are serious, and both can result in death or disability. There is, however, a higher death rate associated with hemorrhagic stroke. Remember, hemorrhagic stroke is caused by bleeding. In addition to reducing the blood supply to the brain, it also floods the brain with blood, which puts pressure on the surrounding brain tissue and further interferes with brain function. According to the AHA, about half of the victims of cerebral hemorrhage die from the increased pressure on their brains. Those who survive hemorrhagic stroke do, however, have a better recovery rate than survivors of ischemic stroke.

Q: Why is that?

A: In ischemic stroke, the damage is caused solely by the death of brain cells. In hemorrhagic stroke, much of the damage is caused by increased pressure on the brain. While brain cells cannot regenerate, pressure on the brain can be diminished.

Q: Who is more likely to have a hemorrhagic stroke?

A: Generally, younger people are more likely to have hemorrhagic strokes than older people. In fact, about half of all strokes in younger people are hemorrhagic. In contrast, only 20 to 25 percent of strokes in older people are hemorrhagic; the majority are ischemic in origin.

Q: Is there any explanation for this?

A: Yes, and it deals with the very nature of stroke. While even the term implies a sudden event, stroke is usually the result of a long-term congenital or chronic condition. In younger people, congenital conditions like vessel malformations are often the cause of stroke; in older people, chronic conditions like atherosclerosis and high blood pressure are often the culprits. In other words, an age-group's tendency toward a certain type of stroke can be explained largely by risk factors. We'll look at those risk factors in detail in the next chapter.

Q: Are there any warning signs for stroke?

A: There certainly are. Note the following: a sudden weakness, numbness or paralysis in your face, arm or leg, particularly on one side of the body; a sudden dimness or blurring of vision, particularly in one eye; an inability to speak or understand spoken language; a sudden, severe headache; unexplained dizziness, unsteadiness or falling; or sudden unconsciousness. Anyone experiencing any of these may be having a stroke and should seek medical attention immediately.

Q: I know someone who experienced several of those warning signs but was fine several hours later. Is that possible?

A: Yes. What you've described is a **transient ischemic attack (TIA)**, or ministroke. A TIA occurs when a narrowed artery, clot or some other foreign material temporarily blocks blood flow to the brain, causing strokelike symptoms. Unlike a full-fledged stroke, however, blood flow in a TIA quickly returns to normal, and all symptoms disappear within 24 hours.

Q: Is that what's meant by the term "minor stroke"?

A: No. A minor stroke lasts longer than a TIA and may produce some lasting effects. There are two types of minor stroke. The first, **reversible ischemic neurological deficit (RIND)**, occurs when the stroke-like symptoms last longer than 24 hours but leave only minor deficits. The second, **partially reversible ischemic neurological deficit (PRIND)**, occurs when the symptoms last more than three days and produce minor dysfunction.

WARNING SIGNS OF STROKE

- Sudden weakness, numbness or paralysis in face, arm or leg (particularly on one side of the body)

- Sudden dimness or blurring of vision (particularly in one eye)

- Inability to speak or understand spoken language

- Sudden, severe headache

- Unexplained dizziness, unsteadiness or falls

- Sudden unconsciousness

Q: That doesn't sound too bad, but I'd like to avoid stroke altogether. Can stroke be prevented?

A: To some degree, yes. While there is no surefire way to predict when a blood vessel might rupture or when a blood clot might develop and block a crucial artery, the risks of either occurrence can be reduced. If aneurysms and blood-vessel malformations are detected, for example, they can be surgically corrected. And various precautions and lifestyle changes can help prevent the development of blood clots or lessen the severity of other conditions that put you at risk for stroke. In short, the best way to prevent a stroke is to reduce your stroke risk factors.

3 RISK ANALYSIS

Q: What are the risk factors for stroke?

A: Because stroke is a cerebrovascular disorder, it has many of the same risk factors as heart disease and other cardiovascular disorders, including **hypertension** (high blood pressure), atherosclerosis, diabetes and smoking, as well as sex, age and heredity. In fact, heart disease itself is a major risk factor. Stroke also carries its own risk factors, including transient ischemic attacks (TIAs) and a personal history of prior stroke.

In general, stroke risks can be classified into three types: (1) those that can't be changed or controlled, (2) those that can't be changed but can be controlled to some extent, and (3) those that can be either changed or controlled. Some of the risks in the latter group—for example, diet, physical inactivity and weight—are actually secondary risk factors—factors that do not place a person at risk for stroke, but rather at risk for developing other stroke risk factors.

Q: Do multiple risk factors increase the chances of having a stroke?

A: Yes, more risk factors means greater overall risk. That's why it's important to know your risk factors and eliminate or control as many as possible. Rest assured, however, that being at increased risk for stroke does not mean you will definitely have a stroke, just that you are more likely to have a stroke than someone who is not at increased risk.

UNCONTROLLABLE RISK FACTORS

Q: What are the uncontrollable risk factors?

A: Unfortunately, there are quite a few. They include:

- age
- sex
- race
- **sickle-cell disease**
- diabetes
- a tendency toward migraine headaches
- a personal or family history of stroke.

In addition, it appears that season, climate and geographic area may also contribute to stroke risk.

Personal History

Q: Can we take a closer look at these uncontrollable risks, beginning with age?

A: Of course. As we've already seen, older people have a greater risk of ischemic stroke than younger people. And since ischemic stroke is the most common type of stroke, older people are at greater risk of stroke in general. In fact, nearly three-quarters of all strokes occur in people 65 or older. According to the American Heart Association, the risk of stroke in people ages 65 to 74 is about 1 percent a year. That risk more than doubles with each decade after 65. And that doesn't take into consideration the addition of other risk factors.

Q: Like family history, race and sex?

A: Yes. Some of the very things that define you as a person—your age, sex, race and genetic makeup— can put you at risk for stroke. Although the precise role of genetics in stroke risk has not yet been determined (some studies have found a direct link between a family's history of stroke and stroke risk; others have not), family history is clearly a factor in other stroke risks. Examples of genetic factors are sickle-cell disease, diabetes and hypertension. Race is also an important genetic stroke risk factor. For example, African Americans are about 60 percent more likely to have a stroke than whites. African American men have the highest risk, since the incidence of stroke is 19 percent higher for men in general, according to the American Heart Association.

Q: Why is that?

A: No one knows for sure, but experts think it might have something to do with the prevalence of other risk factors in both groups. Men, for example, have a higher frequency of heart disease than women, and African Americans have a higher frequency of hypertension, sickle-cell disease and other stroke risk factors than do whites.

Diseases and Conditions

Q: What is sickle-cell disease?

A: Sickle-cell disease is an inherited disorder in which the red blood cells develop a curved, sickle shape. These misshapen cells are fragile. They can break up, resulting in **anemia**, or they can become stuck in small blood vessels, blocking the blood flow and causing pain. If they block the blood vessels that lead to the brain, a stroke may result.

Q: Who gets sickle-cell disease?

A: The disease most often strikes people of negroid descent, but it can also affect Hispanics from the Caribbean, Central America and South America, as well as non-Hispanic people from Turkey, Greece, Italy and the Middle East.

Q: Is stroke a common complication of sickle-cell disease?

A: While stroke is listed as a "relatively infrequent" complication in the U.S. Department of Health and Human Services' Clinical Practice Guideline for sickle-cell disease, sickle-cell disease is the most common cause of stroke in children, according to *The American Heart Association Family Guide to Stroke Treatment, Recovery and Prevention.* One in 14 people with sickle-cell disease eventually has a stroke. And the average age for a child with sickle-cell disease to have a stroke is seven years.

Q: Is there any treatment for sickle-cell disease?

A: There is, but it does not reduce stroke risk: People with sickle-cell disease are often given antibiotics to prevent infections, and a new drug, hydroxyurea, shows promise for reducing both pain and the need for transfusions. But hydroxyurea, which is currently used to treat various forms of cancer, has not yet been approved for the treatment of sickle-cell disease, so as yet there are no medical treatments that reduce stroke risk or control the disease.

Q: There are treatments that control diabetes, however. So how can it be an uncontrollable risk factor for stroke?

A: Even though diabetes can be controlled, it still puts its victims at increased risk for stroke. In fact, one-fifth of stroke sufferers are diabetic. But while diabetics are at greater risk of stroke than nondiabetic people, those who have the condition under control are at less risk of suffering a stroke than those who do not. They also have a better prognosis if they do suffer a stroke.

Q: **You also mentioned migraine headaches. How do they increase stroke risk?**

A: That's a tricky question, or rather a question with a tricky answer. Researchers have found a definite link between migraine headaches and stroke, but they're not exactly sure what that link indicates.

In a study reported in the *British Medical Journal* in 1993, researchers compared the migraine histories of 212 stroke victims with a control group of the same number and found a significant association between migraines and strokes in women under 45, particularly if they had a history of both migraines and smoking. A smaller study, reported at the American Heart Association's 1994 stroke meeting, confirmed those findings. In that study, French researchers found that women under 45 who suffer migraines have a risk of ischemic stroke four times greater than those who do not have migraines. If they smoke, that risk rises to 10 times more.

Q: **Is this risk limited to young women?**

A: That's difficult to say. Neither of the above-mentioned studies found a link between migraines and stroke in older women or in men, but a study presented at the 1991 meeting of the American Heart Association found that men who get migraine headaches are twice as likely to have a stroke as those who do not. Results of a Harvard University study of 22,000 male physicians, published in the *Archives of Neurology* (February 1995), appear to confirm the 1991 study. The Harvard study found that the men who suffered from migraine headaches were 80 percent more likely to have any type of stroke and twice as likely to have an ischemic stroke.

Q: Do these researchers believe migraines actually cause stroke?

A: Not at all. They say migraines simply indicate a possible increase in stroke risk. Migraines appear to be a marker for some other condition that directly increases the risk of stroke. Obviously, further research is needed to identify the connection.

Season, Climate and Geography

Q: Speaking of connections, how is stroke related to season, climate and geographic area?

A: Once again, we're dealing with general observations that cannot be fully explained. Researchers have found that stroke, in general, is more common during periods of extreme temperatures, while stroke caused by subarachnoid hemorrhage is more common among men in late fall and among women in the spring.

Q: Why is that?

A: No one is certain, but it could have something to do with changes in weather patterns or weather-related changes in people's behavior. A 1993 Northwestern University Medical School study that identified the seasonal risk in subarachnoid hemorrhage suggests that weather changes, at least in colder climates, are an important factor for men.

Researchers analyzed the records of 1,487 Connecticut residents who suffered subarachnoid hemorrhages and found that 40 percent of the men studied suffered strokes in November and December—often within 72 hours of a major change in the weather. These changes, which included falling barometers, plunging temperatures and precipitation, seemed to have no effect on women, however. Women were more likely to have strokes in April and May.

Researchers speculate that people may change their behaviors when the seasons turn, somehow increasing their risks for hemorrhagic stroke. In men, they said, the increased risk may be due in part to the cold, which can raise blood pressure and make blood thicker. Either occurrence could increase damage to a weak artery wall and cause the artery rupture.

Q: That makes sense. So is stroke more common in colder geographic regions?

A: Actually, stroke is more common in the southeastern United States, where the weather is relatively warm. The so-called **Stroke Belt** is comprised of Alabama, Arkansas, Georgia, Indiana, Kentucky, Louisiana, Mississippi, North Carolina, South Carolina, Tennessee and Virginia.

Q: Does the warmer weather make people in this region more susceptible to stroke?

A: It might. As we said earlier, extremes in temperature have been linked to increased stroke risks. But no one knows for sure why strokes are more common in the Southeast. Among the possible explanations some experts give are the regional diet, high levels of obesity, hypertension and stress, and relatively limited access to health care.

Q: **Is it my imagination, or do these uncontrollable risk factors—geography, weather and conditions like migraine—seem to come with a lot of unknowns?**

A: It's not your imagination. Stroke is a complicated disorder that involves two complex body systems —the nervous system and the vascular system. And both of these systems can be affected by a variety of factors. With so many factors involved, it's natural that some aren't completely understood. Fortunately, we know more about the risk factors that can be partially or fully controlled.

PARTIALLY CONTROLLABLE RISK FACTORS

Q: **What are the partially controllable risk factors?**

A: The list includes some real heavyweights:

- TIAs, or "ministrokes"

- hypertension

- atherosclerosis, often signaled by noises, or **bruits**, in one or both of the **carotid arteries**

- various forms of heart disease, including **arrhythmias** (such as **atrial fibrillation**) and **left ventricular hypertrophy (LVH)**

• high levels of **cholesterol** in the blood

• blood abnormalities, such as a high red-blood-cell count.

Some of these risk factors are serious problems in their own right, and none can simply be eliminated. Fortunately, however, their effects on the body and on stroke risk can be reduced through medications, surgical procedures or lifestyle changes.

TIAs

Q: **Then I definitely need more information on each, starting with TIAs. Refresh my memory. What is a TIA?**

A: A TIA is essentially a little stroke. It occurs when a clot or some other foreign matter temporarily blocks an artery, depriving a part of the brain of vitally necessary blood. By definition, however, the blockage and the stroke symptoms last no longer than 24 hours and result in no permanent damage.

Q: **So it's a pretty strong indicator of stroke risk, isn't it?**

A: It certainly is. More than one-third of the people who have had a TIA ultimately have a stroke. In fact, a person who has had a TIA is nearly 10 times more likely to have a stroke than someone of the same age and sex who hasn't had one.

Q: How can I tell if I've had a TIA?

A: TIA symptoms are very similar to stroke symptoms. They include temporary weakness, clumsiness or loss of feeling in an arm, leg or side of the face, particularly on one side of the body; temporary dimness or loss of vision; temporary loss of speech or difficulty in communicating; dizziness; or loss of consciousness.

Q: But once I've experienced these symptoms, I've had the attack. How can a TIA be a controllable risk factor for stroke?

A: Since a TIA is such a strong predictor of stroke, it may alert its victims to their high risk of stroke and enable their doctors to find and treat whatever underlying problems can be treated.

Q: How are TIAs usually treated?

A: They may be treated with **anticoagulants** or **platelet inhibitors**—drugs often referred to as "blood thinners"—or, if the underlying cause is a buildup of atherosclerotic **plaque** in a carotid artery of the neck, with a surgical procedure known as **carotid endarterectomy**. We'll discuss this procedure in detail later in this chapter.

Hypertension

Q: In the meantime, let's tackle hypertension. You said it is high blood pressure, but what exactly is blood pressure?

A: Blood pressure is the pressure of circulating blood against the walls of the body's arteries and veins, and against the chambers of the heart. There are two measurements—**systolic** and **diastolic**. Systolic pressure, the higher number in a blood-pressure reading, measures blood pressure when the blood's force against the vessel walls is at its greatest strength. Diastolic pressure, the lower number, measures the blood pressure when the heart is in its resting phase.

Q: When is a blood-pressure reading considered to be high?

A: Generally, blood pressure is considered to be high if, over an extended period of time, the systolic pressure is equal to or greater than 140 and/or the diastolic pressure is equal to or greater than 90.

Q: Why is high blood pressure bad?

A: Increased blood pressure means that the heart is working harder than normal to push blood through the vascular system. This puts both the heart and the vessels under great strain. The heart may try to compensate by increasing in size, but an enlarged heart is less, rather than more, effective. The vessels, for their part, may become scarred, hardened and more susceptible to atherosclerosis, which narrows the arteries.

Q: And narrowed arteries reduce blood flow. Is that how hypertension increases stroke risk?

A: It's one way, yes. Reduced blood flow to the brain can cause a stroke. In addition, the narrowed arteries make it easier for a clot or other foreign matter in the bloodstream to become lodged in an artery and block blood flow. In fact, the fatty deposits atherosclerosis leaves on artery walls can themselves break off and lodge in an artery.

Hypertension can also increase the risk for hemorrhagic stroke by weakening the blood-vessel walls and making them more vulnerable to rupture.

Q: Sounds like hypertension is a pretty strong risk factor! Is it common?

A: Very. It's estimated that one in four American adults has high blood pressure. And the percentage is even higher among African Americans and people over 65 years of age.

Q: What causes hypertension?

A: In between 90 and 95 percent of the cases, the cause is unknown. Fortunately, however, it is not necessary to know the cause to treat and control hypertension.

Q: Does controlling hypertension reduce stroke risk?

A: It certainly does.

Q: Good. So how is hypertension controlled?

A: Lifestyle changes, medications and a combination of the two can be used to lower blood pressure. It's up to you and your doctor to find the treatment that works for you.

Q: What kind of lifestyle changes might help lower blood pressure?

A: By increasing physical activity, limiting alcohol consumption, maintaining appropriate weight and reducing sodium in the diet, people with mild hypertension may lower their blood pressures. If these changes don't work by themselves, they may be recommended in conjunction with an antihypertensive medication.

Q: You said "an antihypertensive medication." I take it there is more than one kind available?

A: Yes. There are several major classes of antihypertensives, each of which works in a different way. **Diuretics**, for example, rid the body of excess sodium and fluids, while beta blockers slow the heart rate and reduce the production of an enzyme that increases blood vessels' resistance to blood flow. Other classes of antihypertensives include sympathetic nerve inhibitors, which block the brain's message to constrict the blood vessels; vasodilators, which relax the artery walls; angiotensin converting enzyme (ACE) inhibitors, which interfere with constriction; and calcium antagonists or calcium channel blockers, which reduce the heart rate and relax blood vessels.

Atherosclerosis

Q: **Sounds like there are plenty to choose from. Do any of them work against atherosclerosis?**

A: Not directly. But controlling hypertension is one way to keep atherosclerosis in check, since high blood pressure contributes to atherosclerosis.

Q: **What actually causes atherosclerosis?**

A: That question brings us back into "unknown" territory. We know that hypertension, serum cholesterol levels and smoking contribute to atherosclerosis, but the actual cause of the disease is unknown. Some experts think it begins when the inner lining of an artery becomes injured in some way, allowing fats, cholesterol and other substances to become deposited on the artery walls; others believe it is caused by either an increase of muscle in the vessel walls or a genetic defect.

Q: **I know we've been over this before, but how exactly does atherosclerosis contribute to stroke risk?**

A: Plaque, the fatty buildup on the artery walls, thickens, hardens and narrows those walls. Once an artery is narrowed, it becomes easier for a clot or piece of foreign matter (even a piece of atherosclerotic plaque) to become lodged in it, blocking blood flow. If this buildup occurs in one of the blood vessels leading to the brain, it greatly increases the risk of stroke.

Q: Is there any way to tell if this has happened?

A: Yes, when the buildup is in a carotid artery of the neck. When carotid arteries are narrowed, they make a swooshing sound called a *bruit* (which is French for "sound") that can be detected with a stethoscope. This sound is considered a very strong risk factor for stroke; it indicates that a substantial narrowing, or **stenosis**, of the carotid artery has already occurred.

Q: Is there any way to remove this buildup?

A: There is a surgical procedure, carotid endarterectomy, which can be used to enlarge the artery opening or replace a portion of the artery.

Q: Isn't that procedure used to treat some TIAs?

A: It is. TIAs often occur in people with substantial carotid stenosis. In fact, TIAs are often signs of severe carotid stenosis.

Q: So carotid endarterectomy is a preventive measure?

A: It can be. It can also be used to restore blood flow and prevent further blockages in people who have already had strokes.

Q: What does the procedure entail?

A: Basically, the surgeon opens the carotid artery and either removes the plaque and closes the artery back up or replaces that portion of the artery with another vein or a Dacron replacement. But the procedure is not as simple as it sounds. Blood flow through the artery must be rerouted before the plaque is removed, so the surgeon constructs a bypass around the obstructed area of the artery. If the bypass is to be permanent, he may cut away the blocked section of the artery. If the bypass is to be temporary, he must repair the artery and restore blood flow after the plaque is removed. In either case, when the blood is rerouted, the surgeon must be careful to assure that clots don't enter the blood flow.

Q: What happens if they do?

A: They can cause the very thing the surgery is designed to prevent—stroke.

Q: Does that happen often?

A: Three major studies reported in 1991 found that the rates of stroke, other complications or death were between 5.5 and 7.5 percent in people who underwent the surgery. Medical centers that have expertise in the procedure may have lower rates, however. Experts say the procedure should be performed at centers with a complication rate below 3 percent. While that still may sound high—for some people, it is far lower than the risk of stroke without surgery.

Q: Is the surgery effective?

A: Yes and no. For some people, the surgery is clearly effective; for others it's clearly ineffective. And for another class of people its effectiveness is unknown.

Q: Give me the definites first. When is carotid endarterectomy effective and when is it not?

A: The procedure has been proven to reduce the incidence of TIA and stroke in people who have had one or more TIAs and whose carotid arteries have severe blockages—70 percent or more. It is not effective in people whose arteries have mild blockages—less than 30 percent. Its effectiveness is also questionable in people with moderate blockages—between 30 and 60 percent— who have not had TIAs or strokelike symptoms.

Q: For which group is its effectiveness unknown?

A: Conflicting research makes it difficult to determine if endarterectomy is effective in people who have severe blockage of the carotid but who have no symptoms. The three 1991 studies found no benefit, but a study completed in late 1994 found that endarterectomy cut stroke risk in half in people who had carotid blockages of 60 percent or more but no symptoms. The procedure appears to be more beneficial for men than for women, however. The 1994 study, published in the May 10, 1995, *Journal of the American Medical Association,* found that it reduced the risk of stroke in men by 69 percent but in women by only 16 percent.

Q: Why is that?

A: No one is certain. It could be that the women in the study had fewer risk factors to begin with and were simply less likely to suffer strokes. It could also have something to do with the smaller size of women's arteries.

Q: The procedure seems to be controversial. Even medical studies don't agree on when and for whom it is appropriate. So what's the bottom line? Who should undergo this procedure?

A: That's a tough question. It may be easier to identify who should *not* have the procedure. Carotid endarterectomy is not for everybody. It is ineffective in people with mild artery blockages and no symptoms, and its effectiveness is questionable in people with moderate blockages and no symptoms. And, while it appears to be beneficial in people with severe blockages whether they have symptoms or not, it is not recommended for anyone with conditions that might increase its complication rate. This includes people with coronary artery disease and uncontrolled hypertension. In these people and certain others, the risks of the procedure may outweigh the benefits. Because of these risks and uncertainty, anyone for whom an endarterectomy is recommended should get at least one independent, second opinion before undergoing the procedure.

Q: Are there other treatments or procedures recommended to people who have blocked carotid arteries?

A: Yes. Platelet inhibitors, such as aspirin, or anti-coagulants, such as **warfarin**, may be used to prevent blood from clotting; antihypertensives and life-style changes may be used to control hypertension; and lifestyle changes may be recommended to keep athero-sclerotic carotid-artery disease in check. These recommendations will probably include directions to stop smoking and reduce the amount of fat and cholesterol in the diet.

In terms of procedures, research is under way to determine if **balloon angioplasty**, a procedure now commonly used to clear blocked coronary arteries, may be effective in clearing the carotid artery. The procedure, which is not yet commonly used in carotid-artery disease, involves inserting a long, balloon-tipped catheter into the patient's groin, then guiding it, via x-rays, to the partially blocked artery. The balloon is then inflated to enlarge the artery opening. Angioplasty would be less expensive and less invasive than carotid endarterectomy, but more research is needed to determine how the procedure compares with endarterectomy in safety and effectiveness.

Heart Disease

Q: While we're talking about the cardiovascular system, could you explain how heart disease factors into stroke risk?

A: Certainly. As you know, the heart is responsible for pumping oxygen-rich blood through the arteries and blood vessels and, ultimately, through the body—including the brain. Any problem that affects the heart's ability to do its job or creates problems for the vascular system may affect the amount of blood received by the brain. Unfortunately, the heart is susceptible to a number of problems, some (like heart failure) that directly affect blood flow, causing hypoperfusion, and others that create **embolisms** that travel to and lodge in the arteries serving the brain. In either case, these problems can cause stroke. In fact, it is estimated that some form of heart disease is responsible for 20 percent of all ischemic strokes. It easily doubles stroke risk.

Q: **What problems in particular might lead to the creation of embolisms?**

A: Heart attacks, valvular heart disease and arrhythmias can all generate embolisms, as can the presence of atherosclerosis in the aorta (the artery that receives oxygenated blood from the heart and distributes it to the body) or the coronary arteries, which provide blood to the heart itself.

Q: **I understand how atherosclerosis can generate embolisms, but what about the first three problems you just mentioned?**

A: Heart attacks, as you recall, are caused by clots; they decrease the heart's ability to supply sufficient blood to the body. This is also the case with valvular heart disease and arrhythmias. Artificial heart valves, used to replace valves damaged by disease, have been known to generate clots. And arrhythmias like atrial fibrillation sometimes affect the heart's ability to fully empty itself of blood, allowing it to pool in the heart's chambers and clot. Unfortunately, both heart attacks and valve disorders can lead to arrhythmias in addition to causing problems of their own.

Q: What type of arrhythmia is atrial fibrillation?

A: Atrial fibrillation is the irregular contraction of the walls of the heart's upper chamber (atrium). In some instances, the atria fail to empty completely, which can allow blood to pool and clot. Atrial fibrillation occurs in 2 percent of the population and in 5 percent of those over 60.

Q: How big of a risk factor for stroke is it?

A: Atrial fibrillation is associated with between 6 and 24 percent of ischemic strokes and 50 percent of cardioembolic strokes—those in which the embolism originated in the heart. The stroke rate for people with atrial fibrillation is about 5 percent a year. Experts say the figure is so high because many people with atrial fibrillation also have carotid artery stenosis, hypertension and diabetes.

Q: How is atrial fibrillation treated?

A: Two kinds of medications may be used to treat arrhythmias like atrial fibrillation—the first controls the heart's rhythm by reducing or increasing the speed of the heartbeat; the second reduces the risk of embolism development. As you might guess, it is the latter kind of medication—primarily the anticoagulant warfarin or the platelet inhibitor aspirin—that is touted as a way to reduce stroke risk.

Q: How effective are these drugs?

A: Studies conducted during the past few years suggest that warfarin can reduce the risk of stroke in people with atrial fibrillation by almost 70 percent. But the drug increases the risk of internal bleeding. Aspirin, a less risky but less effective option, has been shown to reduce stroke risk in people with atrial fibrillation by between 22 and 42 percent.

Q: Are these drugs used to treat other heart problems that can cause stroke?

A: They can be. In general, anticoagulants are prescribed to prevent clots after a heart attack; anticoagulants are also given to people with valvular heart disease and people who have artificial heart valves. Artificial-heart-valve recipients may also be treated with platelet inhibitors.

Q: What about left ventricular hypertrophy?

A: Left ventricular hypertrophy (LVH) is a condition in which the left ventricle (lower chamber) of the heart is enlarged. LVH is common among older people with high blood pressure and has long been suspected of increasing the risk for stroke. A study involving the participants of the famed Framingham Heart Study recently confirmed that suspicion. The study, published in the July 6, 1994, *Journal of the American Medical Association,* measured the hearts of 1,230 elderly people and tracked their history of stroke and other cerebrovascular events. Researchers found that the participants with the largest left ventricles were nearly three times more likely to suffer strokes than those with the smallest left ventricles.

LVH is often the result of the heart's attempt to compensate for the strain caused by hypertension. Treating hypertension can relieve the strain and stop the ventricle from getting any bigger.

Q: Are there any other ways to reduce the stroke risk created by heart disease?

A: Yes. You can work to reduce your risk of heart disease. Keep blood pressure and diabetes under control; don't smoke; maintain your proper weight; increase your level of physical activity; and reduce your dietary intake of fat and cholesterol.

Cholesterol Levels

Q: You've mentioned cholesterol several times. How does it increase stroke risk?

A: Cholesterol does not directly increase the risk of stroke, but it is associated with both atherosclerosis and heart disease. The fatlike substance, which is carried through the bloodstream, is a building block for plaque. When it is present in the blood in high levels, it can deposit itself on artery walls, narrowing the arteries. This contributes to atherosclerosis and heart disease.

Q: Where does this cholesterol come from?

A: Cholesterol is taken in from food and is also produced by the body. In other words, there are two sources: the human liver, which manufactures it, and a diet of animal foods, such as meat, fish, poultry, egg yolks and whole-milk dairy products.

Q: Does reducing consumption of those foods lower blood cholesterol levels?

A: It can. Eating a diet low in cholesterol and saturated fats does help reduce the risk of high blood cholesterol, but dietary restrictions don't always lower blood cholesterol to safe levels. There are also medications available to reduce blood cholesterol levels.

Q: Does lowering blood cholesterol levels directly reduce stroke risk?

A: That's a matter of some contention. On the one side, experts agree that lowering blood cholesterol levels reduces the risk for atherosclerosis and heart disease, both strong risk factors for stroke. On the other side, however, no one has been able to prove that lowering blood cholesterol levels actually reduces stroke risk. In fact, an analysis of 13 studies, reported in the July 15, 1993, *Annals of Internal Medicine,* found that lowering total blood cholesterol levels through diet and medication did not reduce stroke risk in middle-aged men. Still, most experts recommend that blood cholesterol levels be monitored and controlled to help control atherosclerosis and heart disease.

Blood Disorders

Q: Didn't you say there are blood disorders that increase the risk of stroke?

A: Yes. The most well known is **polycythemia**, and it involves an abnormal increase in the number of red blood cells. Red blood cells thicken the blood, affecting its ability to flow and making it more likely to clot.

Stroke risk may also be heightened if the blood contains high levels of **fibrinogen**, a protein used in the blood-clotting process. Studies indicate that high levels of fibrinogen change the viscosity, or thickness, of blood. It may promote clotting and encourage platelets to cluster.

Q: Let me guess. Are these conditions treated with blood thinners?

A: They certainly are. Platelet inhibitors and other medications that help the blood flow smoothly keep polycythemia in check and can reduce the blood viscosity caused by high levels of fibrinogen, but experts say there is a need for a medication that can consistently lower fibrinogen levels.

CONTROLLABLE RISK FACTORS

Q: But aren't there also risk factors that can be totally controlled or eliminated?

A: There certainly are. In fact, we've already discussed quite a few of them. Many of the controllable risk factors are considered secondary risk factors—they contribute indirectly to a person's stroke risk. They do so by increasing his other, primary stroke-risk factors.

Among these secondary risk factors are obesity, physical inactivity, drug abuse and an excessive intake of alcohol. Smoking is both a primary and a secondary risk factor. In addition to increasing stroke risk alone, it exacerbates blood pressure, atherosclerosis and heart disease. Smoking also increases the risk of stroke in women taking oral contraceptives.

Smoking

Q: **Since smoking seems to be the most serious, let's start with it. How does smoking increase stroke risk?**

A: It works in three ways: The nicotine present in cigarettes causes the heart and blood vessels to constrict, which increases blood pressure and heart rate. And carbon monoxide, a by-product of smoking, decreases the amount of oxygen available, making the heart work harder. Finally, smoking causes blood platelets to become stickier and cluster together, increasing the buildup of plaque on artery walls.

Q: **So what is smoking's overall effect on stroke risk?**

A: This single risk factor—smoking—increases stroke risk by 40 percent in men and 60 percent in women. And women who smoke and take oral contraceptives are 22 times more likely to have a stroke than those who do neither.

Q: Do oral contraceptives pose a danger on their own?

A: Birth-control pills containing high levels of estrogen and progestin are associated with an increased stroke risk. The risk associated with the newer, low-dose oral contraceptives is not as great, however. Studies have shown that the risk of stroke decreases as the hormone dose decreases. But while some studies indicate that the use of low-dose contraceptives does not significantly increase the risk of stroke, others indicate that it does. All studies have found, however, that the risk of stroke is higher when users of any contraceptive—high dose or low—smoke.

The bottom line is that women who smoke should not use oral contraceptives, and women who use oral contraceptives should not smoke. Better yet, women—and men for that matter—should not smoke at all.

Q: What about people who do smoke? Does their risk of stroke decrease if they stop?

A: Absolutely. The Framingham Heart Study found that after five years of not smoking, the risk of stroke in former smokers was equal to that of those who had never smoked. Another study indicates that the risk may disappear even faster. Data from the Nurses' Health Study, reported in the January 13, 1993, *Journal of American Medicine,* found that it took former women smokers only two to four years to reduce their stroke risk to that of women who never smoked. And, the study found, the decline in risk occurred regardless of the age at which the women started smoking or the number of cigarettes they smoked.

Secondary Risk Factors

Q: Getting back to the truly secondary risks, what risk factors does obesity increase?

A: Obesity—weighing 20 percent more than your ideal body weight—increases the risk of diabetes, heart disease and hypertension. Being overweight places heavy demands on the body for more insulin, contributes to insulin resistance and increases strain on the heart. This increases the risk of diabetes and heart disease, which are both major risk factors for stroke.

Recent studies have shown that it's not just the presence of extra weight but also its distribution on the body that affects heart-disease risk. Weight that is carried around the waist apparently poses the most danger. The risk of developing heart disease is significantly increased in men whose waist measurements exceed their hip measurements and in women whose waist measurements are more than 80 percent of their hip measurements.

Q: Are the risks for heart disease and diabetes reduced when excess weight is lost?

A: Yes. Losing weight reduces strain on the body and reduces the risks of developing heart disease and diabetes, and indirectly, stroke.

Q: I know weight loss depends a great deal on diet. Does diet have any other effects on stroke?

A: It might. At least three types of food—fish, fruits and vegetables—have been linked to low stroke risks. A study published in the February 1994 issue of *Stroke* found that men who consumed at least one portion of fish a week had about half the risk of stroke as men who did not eat that amount of fish. And new data from the Framingham Heart Study, published in the April 12, 1995, *Journal of the American Medical Association,* indicates that for each increment of three servings of fruits and vegetables a day, middle-aged men may be able to reduce their stroke risk by 22 percent. So diet may be important independent of its effect on obesity.

Q: What about physical inactivity?

A: Physical inactivity can contribute to obesity and increased blood cholesterol levels, thus increasing the risk of heart disease and hypertension, primary stroke-risk factors. Remember, the heart is a muscle, and like other muscles, it can be strengthened with exercise. Exercise can slow the heart rate and reduce the pulse, both of which are good for the heart. It can also reduce blood pressure and aid in weight loss.

Q: What kind of exercise is best for heart health?

A: To promote cardiovascular fitness, experts have for years recommended aerobic exercise—vigorous activities, such as running and aerobic dance, that increase the body's need for and utilization of oxygen—for at least 20 minutes three or four times a week. But recent studies indicate that even moderate activities like walking, gardening and housework can be beneficial to the heart. The latest guidelines recommend 30 minutes of moderate activity five times a week.

Moderate activity may also have a direct effect on stroke. A Yale study reported in 1995 found that middle-aged men who walked a mile every day decreased their stroke risk by almost 50 percent. This exercise appeared to reduce stroke risk in and of itself—the benefits of exercise persisted even after the researchers controlled for other stroke risk factors. Still, you should check with your doctor before significantly increasing your level of physical activity.

Q: **I don't need a doctor to know I shouldn't abuse drugs. But how does drug abuse increase the risk of stroke?**

A: Intravenous drug abuse increases the risk of developing embolisms. And stimulants and hallucinogens, such as cocaine, LSD and amphetamines, increase blood pressure and narrow blood vessels, increasing the risk of both ischemic and hemorrhagic stroke.

Q: **What about alcohol? I keep reading that it's good for the heart. Is moderate drinking a problem in stroke?**

A: No. In fact, moderate drinking may be good for the cerebrovascular system. A 1993 study reported in *Stroke* found that moderate drinkers have a lower risk of stroke than either abstainers or heavy drinkers. But heavy drinking has an adverse effect on stroke risk.

Q: **What effect is that?**

A: Consuming too much alcohol can elevate blood pressure and cause arrhythmia and other heart problems. And binge drinking—exceeding the amount of alcohol you normally consume—can trigger strokes, particularly in people with arrhythmias. This is because intoxicated individuals have rapid pulses that can dislodge blood clots and carry them to the brain.

Q: So how much is too much?

A: Binge drinking in any amount is unhealthy. Otherwise, the American Heart Association recommends limiting consumption to no more than one ounce of pure alcohol a day. This translates into two ounces of 100-proof spirits, eight ounces of wine or 24 ounces of beer.

Q: We seem to have covered all the risk factors you mentioned. Is there anything else I should know about stroke risks?

A: Yes. Although some risks are more serious than others, it's the combination of risks that actually determines how likely you are to have a stroke. You've seen how stroke risk increases when smoking is combined with taking oral contraceptives. Other combinations can also increase stroke risk significantly. Therefore, it's wise to be aware of your risks and do whatever you can to reduce them. That's the best way to prevent a stroke.

Q: With that in mind, could you sum up how to reduce those risks?

A: Certainly. Have regular checkups to monitor blood pressure, diabetes, heart disease or any other condition you may have; control those conditions the best you can with medication or lifestyle changes; maintain an appropriate body weight; exercise; don't smoke; eat a balanced, low-fat, low-cholesterol diet (one that includes fish, fruits and vegetables); don't drink excessively or abuse drugs; and know the warning signs of stroke.

4 IS IT STROKE?

Q: Refresh my memory. What are the warning signs of stroke?

A: Several warning signs indicate stroke: sudden weakness, numbness or paralysis of the face, arm or leg on one side of the body; sudden dimness or loss of vision, particularly in one eye; loss of the ability to speak or difficulty understanding what others say; sudden, severe headaches, which may be accompanied by nausea and vomiting; unexplained dizziness, unsteadiness or falls; or unconsciousness.

Q: Do these symptoms mean that a stroke is in progress?

A: Not necessarily. You've probably noticed that many of them bear a remarkable resemblance to the symptoms of transient ischemic attack. They may simply indicate that a TIA is in progress. But remember, a TIA is a pretty good predictor of stroke. Further, the mechanics of ischemic stroke and TIAs are so similar that a doctor's diagnosis may be needed to determine which is occurring.

Q: Could these symptoms indicate something other than stroke or TIA?

A: Yes. They could also indicate a seizure, migraine headache, brain tumor or, in the case of facial paralysis, a condition known as Bell's palsy. Again, a medical expert should determine the cause.

Q: In other words, regardless of whether or not these symptoms signal stroke, they signal a visit to the doctor, right?

A: Right. It's difficult for an untrained person to tell what has triggered such symptoms, and many of the possibilities require immediate medical attention. In the case of stroke, prompt diagnosis and treatment may mean the difference between life and death.

Q: How? Doctors can't actually stop a stroke once it's started, can they?

A: No. But they can restore blood flow to the brain and lessen a stroke's damage. That's why it's so important to get medical help as soon as possible after the symptoms occur.

Q: Is there anything a bystander can do to help someone who's experiencing these symptoms, other than making arrangements to get her to a medical facility?

A: Medically, no. Unless the person has stopped breathing or has no pulse, there are no real first-aid measures that can be taken other than immediately calling for emergency help. Simply note whether she is conscious and alert and keep her calm and comfortable until help arrives. Do not give her any food or water; if it is a stroke, her ability to swallow might be impaired.

Q: What happens once the person reaches a hospital?

A: Doctors will monitor her vital signs and treat any problems while they determine whether or not she's had a stroke. If she has had a stroke, they must determine what type of stroke it is, what caused it, where it's located and how serious it is so they can begin treatment.

Q: How do they determine these details?

A: Doctors base their diagnoses on information derived from medical history, a physical examination, blood tests, neurological tests, and tests that examine the brain, blood vessels and heart.

MEDICAL HISTORY

Q: Sounds like a complicated process! I'd like to know a little more about it. Let's say I have strokelike symptoms and I'm taken to the hospital. What would a doctor do first?

A: If you are alert and able to talk, the doctor would probably start by asking you questions about your medical history.

Q: What can that information tell him?

A: Plenty. Think back to the risk factors for stroke and remember that stroke is often caused by long-term, chronic conditions. If, for example, the doctor learns from his interview that you have had TIA symptoms, have high blood pressure and have been smoking for the last 20 years, he'll have some indication that you've suffered an ischemic stroke. He will have to do further testing to make sure but will be well on his way to making a diagnosis.

Q: Does this medical history deal strictly with stroke risks?

A: It shouldn't. The doctor also needs to ask about any other medical conditions that might affect your treatment. If you have hemophilia, for example, certain medications used in treating stroke could be more harmful than helpful. Likewise, the doctor needs to know if you are allergic to any medications or if you are taking any medications that might cause a negative reaction when combined with stroke treatment.

Q: Will the doctor ask anything else?

A: He'll probably want to know the specifics of your symptoms—when they started, how long they lasted, which ones came first and that sort of thing. This can help him determine not only whether you've had a stroke, but also its type, location and time of origination. While some symptoms—weakness, paralysis or loss of sensation on one side of the body, for example—are common to both types of stroke, others clearly indicate one type or the other. Language and communication problems, balance problems and mental confusion usually indicate ischemic stroke, while headaches and loss of consciousness signal hemorrhagic stroke.

Q: **What if my symptoms include speech difficulties? How can the doctor get the answers he needs?**

A: If you're unable to speak or recall the information you've been asked, the doctor may question the family member or friend who accompanied you to the hospital. If you came alone—say, by ambulance, after collapsing on a street or sidewalk—the hospital will probably contact your family and your own doctor, if known, while the attending doctor continues with other diagnostic procedures.

PHYSICAL EXAMINATION

Q: What will he start with?

A: Usually a physical exam. The doctor will check your breathing, temperature, pulse and blood pressure. He will listen to your heart to see if he hears anything unusual; he may also put his stethoscope to your neck to listen for carotid bruits. His exam will probably also include a look at your eyes (blood may appear there in hemorrhagic stroke) and a series of blood tests.

Q: What kind of blood tests?

A: Your blood can tell the doctor a lot about you, so the tests he orders will depend on what he wants to know. If he wants to know about your blood's ability to flow, he may order tests that measure its viscosity or the number of red blood cells it contains; if he wants to know about its clotting ability, he may opt for tests that measure the amount of fibrinogen or number of platelets in the blood or the amount of time it takes for the blood to clot. In addition, he may order standard tests to measure fats and sugar in the blood.

NEUROLOGICAL TESTS

Q: Will the exam include any other tests?

A: The doctor will probably also perform a series of simple neurological tests to determine how, or if, your brain has been affected by whatever condition has caused your symptoms.

Q: What do these tests entail?

A: Primarily a lot of questions. The doctor needs to know if you're conscious and oriented and if your memory has been affected. He may ask you if you know who and where you are, if you remember what happened to you or if you remember where you were born. He also needs to determine if your visual and thinking skills are intact; he may point to certain objects in the room and ask you what they are, hold up a certain number of fingers and ask you how many are there or ask you simple mathematical problems.

Some of these questions will be so simplistic that you may feel they are an insult to your intelligence. This is one case, however, where it's good to add insult to injury. If you do feel insulted, chances are your basic thinking, communication and memory skills have not been seriously affected by stroke. If those skills were affected, those seemingly easy questions would be quite difficult and very frustrating.

Q: **I'm beginning to see how widespread stroke's effects can be. Does the doctor look for anything else during the neurological exam?**

A: Yes. While the doctor is questioning you, he will monitor your ability to understand, process and respond to speech. He may ask you to read or write a paragraph or repeat something he has said. He'll also watch your level of alertness and the movement of your eyes. At some point during the exam, you may be asked to stand up and walk, so the doctor can watch your gait; or you may be asked to perform simple physical tasks that test your strength and coordination. The doctor may also check your reflexes and test your ability to feel heat, cold and other sensations.

Q: **So what happens next?**

A: By the time the doctor has completed the physical and neurological exams, he should have a pretty good idea whether or not you've had a stroke. If he thinks you have, his next goal is to finalize that diagnosis and pinpoint the cause and location so he can begin treatment.

Q: Why does he have to go through all that rigmarole? Why doesn't he just start treatment?

A: Because the treatment for stroke varies according to its type. Think for a moment about the two types: In cause, they're almost exact opposites—one stems from a blockage that prevents blood from flowing where it should, the other from a leak that allows blood to flow where it shouldn't. These underlying problems demand different responses. Treatments for hemorrhagic stroke do nothing to help lessen the damage of ischemic stroke, while some of the medications used to treat ischemic stroke could actually worsen hemorrhagic stroke.

Q: I hadn't thought of that. I guess I should let the doctor finish his diagnosis. What will he do next?

A: Test you. Depending on what he suspects to be the problem, the doctor will choose his weapon or weapons from a virtual arsenal of tests designed to help him pinpoint his diagnosis. If, for example, he's unsure about the type of stroke or its location, he may order tests that provide an image or picture of the brain; if he wants to know more about the stroke's effects, he may order tests that measure brain functions; if he wants to know about the vascular problems that have triggered an ischemic stroke, he may order tests that measure blood flow or detect artery blockages. As you might guess, the actual number of tests you may undergo is not written in stone.

BRAIN IMAGING AND FUNCTION TESTS

Q: Let's say the doctor suspects I've had a stroke but isn't exactly sure what type. What kind of tests might he order?

A: He may take the problem by the head, so to speak, and begin with tests that show him what's going on in your brain. A number of imaging tests can help him determine what, if any, physical damage has been done, how it was caused and where it is located.

Q: Imaging tests? Like CAT scans?

A: Yes. In fact, **computerized axial tomography (CAT)**, also called **computerized tomography (CT)**, may be the first test the doctor performs. This fast, painless test, which results in a highly detailed picture of internal body parts, is constructed by a computer from hundreds of x-rays. The picture it creates can be used to help determine if a stroke is hemorrhagic or ischemic in nature and help pinpoint its location.

Q: What exactly can CAT show?

A: While CAT has some limitations, it can be used to confirm the presence of cerebral or subarachnoid hemorrhages, define the location and size of a cerebral hemorrhage and provide information about the location of the aneurysms or blood-vessel malformations that could be causing or have caused a hemorrhagic stroke.

Depending on the stroke's severity, a CAT scan can also define the vascular territory and size of infarcts (areas of dead tissue) in ischemic stroke and show the damage left by old infarcts and hemorrhages.

Q: **That sounds like everything the doctor needs to know. Why is there a need for other tests?**

A: Sometimes there isn't, but a CAT scan is not foolproof. For one thing, it takes some time for ischemic strokes to become visible using CAT. If the test is administered shortly after a stroke has occurred, the problem may not show up on the scan. In addition, CAT gives only indirect evidence of ischemic stroke, showing only the resulting damage. So small ischemic strokes and TIAs may never become visible. And CAT scans miss between 5 and 10 percent of subarachnoid hemorrhages.

Q: **Do other imaging tests provide additional information?**

A: Yes. **Magnetic resonance imaging (MRI)**, which uses magnetic fields and radio-frequency pulses to take images of internal body parts, has some of the same limitations as a CAT scan, including the delay in showing infarcts. But MRI can pick up evidence of smaller injuries and also provides a clearer picture than CAT does, enabling doctors to better identify bleeding, blockages and blood-vessel malformations.

Other imaging tests include **positron emission tomography (PET)**, which creates computer-generated x-ray images of the brain using harmless **radioactive isotopes** injected or inhaled into the body, and **radio-nuclide angiography**, also known as a **nuclear brain scan**, in which a machine similar to a Geiger counter charts the path of radioactive compounds that have been injected into the arm. PET shows the processes in the tissue being studied (in this case, how the brain tissue is using oxygen and glucose) and is useful for localizing lesions, characterizing blood flow and detecting conditions that mimic stroke. Radionuclide angiography shows how the brain is functioning—for example, whether its blood vessels are blocked or if certain areas are damaged.

Q: Any other tests that show the brain's ability to function?

A: Two tests show the brain's electrical activity: the **electroencephalogram (EEG)** and the **evoked response** tests. In an EEG, the electrical impulses transmitted and received by brain cells are collected by electrodes placed on the scalp. Less high-tech are the evoked response tests, which measure how the brain handles different sensory stimuli. In these tests, the doctor literally tries to evoke a response by stimulating the senses. He may flash a light in front of the eyes, make a noise in the ear or electrically stimulate a nerve in an arm or leg; then he monitors the reaction.

WHEN FURTHER TESTING IS NEEDED

Q: At this point, shouldn't the doctor have enough information to make his diagnosis?

A: He might. In fact, depending on the type of stroke you've experienced and the test results, he may have made his diagnosis long ago and be in the process of treating you. Remember, not every stroke patient undergoes every test. And by this point, even though he may have ruled out other possibilities and determined that you have had a stroke, he may not know what type of stroke you've had or what caused it.

Q: Will he be able to find these answers?

A: That depends. Further testing can help him determine if the stroke is hemorrhagic or ischemic in nature—information he must know before beginning treatment. Further testing may also help him pinpoint the cause and location of ischemic stroke. But while he should ultimately be able to determine the type of stroke you've had, there's no guarantee he will find the underlying cause.

Q: Can the doctor treat my stroke without knowing its cause?

A: Yes. As long as the doctor knows what type of stroke you've had, he can treat it using general treatment techniques appropriate to the type of stroke. We'll discuss these techniques in Chapter 5.

Tests to Identify Hemorrhagic Stroke

Q: How can the doctor determine once and for all if the stroke was triggered by a hemorrhage?

A: He will probably start with a second CAT or MRI scan. If these new scans still produce vague results, he can opt for a test known as a **lumbar puncture**, or **spinal tap**. Using a long needle, he'll take a sample of the cerebrospinal fluid from your spinal column. He'll then analyze the sample to see if it contains blood. The presence of blood in the fluid indicates hemorrhagic stroke.

Blood Flow and Artery Tests

Q: Okay. Now how does the doctor try to determine the cause and location of ischemic stroke?

A: That's where the blood flow and artery tests come in. Doctors have a smorgasbord of tests they can use to monitor blood flow and detect stenoses, clots and other blockages. Among the most common are high-tech imaging tests like **magnetic resonance angiography;** various forms of **angiography; ultrasound** and its various forms: **Doppler scanning, transcranial Doppler** and **B-mode imaging; phonoangiography;** and eye tests, such as **ophthalmodynamometry** and **ocular plethysmography.**

Angiography

Q: Can we take those one at a time, starting with magnetic resonance angiography?

A: Certainly. Magnetic resonance angiography is similar to MRI in that it uses magnetic fields and radio waves to create images. In this case, however, the images it creates are of the arteries and veins. The test, which is relatively new, can be performed at the same time as MRI and is less invasive and safer than conventional angiography.

Q: What is conventional angiography?

A: Angiography is the x-ray study of the cardio-vascular system—in this case, the blood vessels. In angiography, an opaque substance or dye is injected into blood vessels to make them visible, then x-rays are taken. The resulting picture is called an **angiogram;** an angiogram of the arteries is known as an **arteriogram.** These pictures show if, or how well, blood is flowing through the arteries and can be used to locate blockages.

Q: You said that magnetic resonance angiography is safer than conventional angiography. What is the danger involved?

A: Angiography is invasive; it carries with it a small risk of injury, infection or allergic reaction.

Ultrasound

Q: What about ultrasound?

A: Ultrasound, which uses sound waves to provide images of internal body parts, is noninvasive and relatively safe. In ultrasound testing, a gel is applied to the skin of the area being studied to reduce friction, then an instrument that records sound waves is passed over the area. The sound waves are translated to an image by means of computer technology.

Ultrasound is often used to detect blockages in the carotid artery. It can show the location and extent of a blockage and, with Doppler scanning techniques, detect how well the blood is flowing.

Q: What exactly is Doppler scanning?

A: Doppler scanning is an ultrasound technique used to monitor the behavior of something that moves, such as blood. It derives information from the difference in the frequency of ultrasonic waves reflected from moving and stationary surfaces. It can be used to measure how fast blood is flowing through an artery and is often used to monitor blood flow through the carotid arteries.

Q: Is it ever used to monitor blood flow in the arteries of the brain?

A: Yes. In fact, that's exactly what transcranial Doppler does. It allows the doctor to see how blood is flowing in the intracranial arteries—those within the cranium, or skull. Often used in place of angiography because it's noninvasive, transcranial Doppler can detect severe stenoses or blockages of the intracranial carotid, the middle cerebral and the vertebrobasilar arteries— three of the major arteries supplying blood to the brain.

Q: And what does B-mode imaging do?

A: B-mode imaging, another form of ultrasound, provides three-dimensional images. It can show an injury to an artery and the severity of damage. It may not, however, show clots or stenoses, so it is often done in conjunction with Doppler testing.

Other Tests

Q: What is phonoangiography?

A: Phonoangiography, also called carotid phonoangiography, is a test that evaluates blood flow by
sound. In carotid phonoangiography, a sensitive micro-
phone is placed on the neck over the carotid arteries to
enable bruits to be heard and located.

Q: I understand the hearing connection, but
how are eyes involved in blood flow?

A: Tiny blood vessels run through the eyes, and many
of these vessels are served by the carotid artery.
By measuring the blood pressure or pulse in the eyes, your
doctor can get a pretty good idea of blood flow in other
small arteries, particularly those served by the carotids.

Q: By this point it seems like the doctor has
examined everything from my brain down
to my smallest blood vessels. Are there any
tests left for him to run?

A: Only if he suspects that the stroke was caused by a
heart problem or that a heart problem may affect
its treatment. Remember, many embolic strokes originate
in the heart. If the doctor suspects that a stroke was
caused by an embolism that formed in or near the heart,
he may order an **electrocardiogram (EKG)**, which
records the electrical activity of the heart. This painless,
noninvasive test can detect a host of cardiac abnormalities
and may help the doctor pinpoint the source of the stroke.

Q: How long will all this testing take?

A: That depends on which and how many tests are ordered. Some take minutes and produce immediate results; others take an hour or longer, plus the time to obtain the results. Sometimes it takes several days to obtain the results from all the tests; in fact, the testing itself can continue for several days. In the case of ischemic stroke, for example, CAT scans may be repeated until the infarct appears.

But even if the diagnosis requires numerous tests and all the details aren't known immediately, your condition itself shouldn't go unattended for long. Remember, stroke is an emergency situation that requires immediate care, and hospital personnel should be aware of this. Your tests will take priority over those of nonemergency patients. And there are steps your doctor can take to slow stroke's damage and prevent further problems before all the results are in. In fact, he may have already begun certain aspects of treatment during the testing phase. We discuss the early treatment of stroke in the next chapter.

5 TREATMENT

Q: I know stroke can't be "cured," so what is the purpose of immediate medical treatment?

A: Twenty or even 10 years ago, the answer to that question would be far different from what it is today. In the not-too-distant past, there was little that doctors could do for stroke victims. The risk factors for and underlying causes of stroke were less well known; technology was less sophisticated; there were fewer medications available and many stroke victims didn't report to their doctors until long after their strokes were over and the damage was done. Consequently, the death rate from stroke was high.

Today, however, there is much doctors can do to stabilize stroke victims, restore blood flow to the brain and prevent complications and future strokes. The death rate has dropped significantly. And research, which is continuing at a rapid pace, may soon make it possible to limit and reverse the damage caused by stroke.

Q: Okay. Let's say I've had a stroke. What will my treatment entail?

A: The first thing the doctor will do is monitor your vital signs to make sure that your airway is clear, that your lungs are functioning properly and that your blood is circulating throughout your body. Your heart will also be monitored, as will your blood sugar, hydration and electrolytes. If problems are detected in any of these areas or if you are suffering from a seizure or other medical emergency, the doctor will concentrate on that before actually beginning to treat you for stroke.

Q: Assuming my vital signs are okay, what will the doctor do to treat the stroke?

A: That depends on the type of stroke. In ischemic stroke the first goal is to improve blood flow to the brain; in hemorrhagic stroke it is to relieve pressure and stop the bleeding.

INITIAL MEDICAL TREATMENT OF ISCHEMIC STROKE

Q: Since ischemic stroke is more common, let's start with it. What will the doctor do to improve blood flow?

A: That, too, depends—this time on the cause of the stroke and its stage or severity. If, for example, the stroke was caused by a clot, the doctor may use blood-thinning drugs to prevent the clot from growing and to facilitate blood flow; if it was caused by a buildup of plaque in the carotid artery, she may opt for a carotid endarterectomy. Initial treatment of a completed stroke differs from treatment of a stroke that is still in progress, and some minor strokes may need little or no emergency medical treatment.

Q: Are there any universal treatments?

A: Yes. Regardless of the cause or the stage of an ischemic stroke, blood pressure must be monitored and controlled.

Blood pressure generally rises during a stroke. Experts believe this is the brain's attempt to get more blood. This temporary elevation may or may not present a problem. If the pressure rises enough to damage brain tissue, cause bleeding in the brain or damage the aorta, kidneys or heart, it must be treated immediately. But the doctor must be careful not to lower pressure too quickly or allow it to drop too low. This can result in **hypotension**, or abnormally low blood pressure, which can actually decrease the amount of blood reaching the brain.

And hypotension, whether induced by antihypertensive medication or occurring naturally, must be treated immediately (usually with saline solution) to prevent further damage to the brain.

In addition, the doctor must monitor and control body temperature. A fever of even one degree can increase brain damage, so the doctor must monitor temperature closely and do what she can to bring it down if it rises. This usually entails administering aspirin or acetaminophen (Tylenol), but if these drugs don't work, the doctor may use a cooling blanket.

Q: Okay, now let's get a little more specific. What if the doctor knows that my stroke is ischemic but hasn't determined what caused it?

A: Generally, if your stroke is still in progress and your condition is getting worse, she will treat you with an anticoagulant, usually **heparin**. This drug, which is administered intravenously, can prevent the formation of additional blood clots, prevent existing clots from getting bigger and enable the blood to flow more freely through narrowed arteries.

Q: When else would heparin be given?

A: Heparin is usually the initial treatment for strokes caused by embolisms that form in or around the heart. In this role and others, it functions not only as first-line treatment but also as a preventive measure: According to *Patient Care*'s August 15, 1994, "Emergency Handbook" article on stroke, up to 25 percent of people whose strokes were caused by a cardiac embolus have a second stroke within two weeks.

Heparin is also a standard initial treatment for strokes caused by severe stenosis of the carotid arteries or stenosis or blockage of the **basilar arteries** or **vertebral arteries**, which also feed the brain.

Because heparin and other anticoagulants can cause hemorrhage, however, they are not used in patients who are at risk for hemorrhage. This includes people who have uncontrolled hypertension, gastrointestinal bleeding or thrombocytopenia, an abnormal blood condition that causes bleeding disorders. The risk of hemorrhage is also high in older people and people in whom stroke has already caused large, deep infarcts (areas of dead brain tissue).

Q: Are any other anticoagulants used in the treatment of stroke?

A: Yes. Warfarin, which we discussed in Chapter 3, is also used to treat ischemic stroke. Unlike heparin, which is administered intravenously and is given short-term, warfarin can be given in pill form and can be used for both short- and long-term treatments. As we've discussed, it is administered in the long-term to people with cardiac problems that could trigger stroke and to people with severely narrowed carotid arteries. It can also be used as a short-term, initial treatment for ischemic stroke. Like heparin, however, it is not given to people at risk for hemorrhage.

Q: What kind of drugs can be given to these people?

A: Platelet inhibitors, or platelet antiaggregants, which we discussed in Chapter 3, can sometimes be used to treat strokes in people for whom anticoagulants are not advised. They are also standard treatment for strokes caused by injuries to or diseases of blood vessels, or abnormal blood conditions that increase the blood's tendency to clot. The most commonly prescribed platelet inhibitors for stroke are aspirin, dipyridamole (Persantine) and **ticlopidine** (Ticlid).

Q: Do you mean the doctor might simply tell me to take two aspirin and call her in the morning?

A: The dose and directions may differ, but aspirin is certainly a major player in the treatment of stroke. In addition to improving blood flow and preventing the recurrence of ischemic stroke, aspirin is believed to lessen the severity of stroke when it does recur. An analysis of patients who had recurrent strokes, reported at the 1994 American Academy of Neurology meeting, found that mild and moderate strokes were more common among those who were on aspirin therapy. (Those who were not taking aspirin experienced more severe strokes.) In addition, aspirin-takers had a lower mortality rate than non-aspirin-takers—only 2.4 percent of them died, compared with 8.1 percent.

Q: But don't some people have a problem taking aspirin?

A: Yes. For them, ticlopidine may be the treatment of choice. This drug, which became available in late 1991, is more effective than aspirin in preventing stroke, but it is more expensive. It also increases the risk of neutropenia, a potentially dangerous drop in the number of white blood cells. Because of this risk, ticlopidine is not universally recommended; it is generally reserved for people who cannot take aspirin.

Q: Are any other types of medications used in the initial treatment of ischemic stroke?

A: Yes and no. The ones we've discussed are the most common currently in use. There are, however, several medications that have been used in the past to treat stroke and may still be used by some doctors. These treatments, which include corticosteroids and barbiturates, are now believed to be, but have not yet been proven, unsuccessful.

On the flip side, a number of new treatments, now in the developmental or testing stages, may revolutionize stroke treatment in the near future. These treatments include **thrombolytic**, or clot-busting, medications as well as **cytoprotective** drugs, which reduce brain-cell injury. We'll discuss these in detail later in this chapter.

Q: What about surgery? Didn't you say carotid endarterectomy can be used to treat stroke?

A: Yes. If the stroke is caused by a blockage or narrowing of a carotid artery, endarterectomy (discussed in Chapter 3) is an option for both treating the stroke and preventing additional strokes. It is most commonly used to treat minor strokes caused by low blood flow from the carotid and to prevent further strokes in people with severe stenosis. Again, this procedure is not for everyone. Make sure you get a second opinion if it is recommended for you.

Q: Is angioplasty an option?

A: Not yet. As it is with stroke prevention, angioplasty is still in its experimental stages for treating stroke.

Q: While we're on the subject of experimental treatments, could you tell me more about thrombolytic drugs?

A: Certainly. Thrombolytic drugs, commonly used to treat heart attacks, are now being viewed as a possible treatment for embolic and thrombotic strokes. Popularly known as "clot busters," these drugs literally break down and dissolve clots. In heart-attack patients, they are used to dissolve the clots that are causing the heart attack, thus ending the attack; in stroke, they would be used to dissolve the clots that are causing the stroke.

This would improve blood flow to the brain and could prevent the development of infarcts, thereby reducing the amount of permanent damage done by the stroke.

Q: How effective are thrombolytic drugs?

A: At least six trials are under way to determine just that. Initial results indicate that thrombolytic therapy may be very promising, if administered early and to the right people. Results of the European Cooperative Acute Stroke Study, released in early 1995, found that treatment with thrombolytic drugs within six hours of the start of stroke symptoms increased by 38 percent the number of stroke survivors who had little or no lasting deficits from their strokes. Another major study, sponsored by the National Institutes of Health, is examining the benefit of thrombolytic treatment administered within 90 minutes of the onset of stroke symptoms. Results of that trial are scheduled to be released sometime in 1995.

Q: What drugs are being tested in these trials?

A: The drugs currently being tested for stroke treatment include streptokinase, urokinase and **tissue plasminogen activator (tPA)**. The latter, a chemical made by the body to remove blood clots when they are no longer necessary to close wounds, appears to be the most promising. It remains active in the body for a shorter time than streptokinase and urokinase and thus reduces the risk of hemorrhage.

Q: So thrombolytic therapy isn't risk-free?

A: No, it's not. That is why it is currently being used only in clinical trials. While thrombolytic drugs show great promise in reducing the damage caused by ischemic strokes, they can trigger bleeding, converting a simple infarct into a cerebral hemorrhage. In fact, nearly 35 percent of a certain subgroup of patients treated with tPA in the European Cooperative Acute Stroke Study died —a death rate 14 percent higher than for patients with equally severe strokes who received a placebo.

These results clearly illustrate that thrombolytic therapy is appropriate only for certain stroke victims—i.e., those whose strokes are ischemic in nature and still in their earliest stages. While the subgroup of patients treated with tPA did receive the drug within six hours of the start of their symptoms, they already had large areas of brain injury visible in CAT scans before the treatment was given.

Q: So the risk increases with time?

A: Yes. The risk is higher the later the drug is given, because blood vessels that have been deprived of oxygen become damaged and prone to rupture. Because of this, and because the drugs can't help prevent damage that has already occurred, thrombolytics must be administered early.

Q: What about the other type of drugs you mentioned, cytoprotective drugs? Are they currently being used?

A: Not widely. Like thrombolytic drugs, cyto-protective drugs are still in the testing—and even development—stages. It may be several years before they are commonly used to treat stroke.

Q: What exactly do cytoprotective drugs do?

A: They literally protect cells (*cyto* is Greek for cell) from damage. Also called *neuroprotective drugs,* because the cells they protect are neurons, or brain cells, these drugs interrupt a chain of chemical reactions that leads to the death of brain cells.

Q: I thought brain cells die because they are deprived of oxygen. What role do these chemical reactions play?

A: That's a good question—one that researchers are now trying to answer. What they have determined so far is that brain-cell damage in stroke apparently has two causes. The first, as you know, is a lack of oxygen and glucose. But there's more to the process than that. The death of brain cells and the creation of an infarct together trigger a chain of chemical interactions that damage and kill brain cells in the tissue surrounding the infarct, an area known as the **penumbra**.

This chain reaction, known as the **glutamate cascade**, is believed to begin after brain cells deprived of oxygen release excessive amounts of a **neurotransmitter** called glutamate into the spaces between the cells. The glutamate binds with molecules on neighboring brain cells, sparking an abnormal movement of calcium ions into the neighboring cells. This creates a buildup of calcium and sodium, which is believed to interfere with the cells' ability to respond to signals from other cells. At the same time, water also accumulates, swelling the cells. Ultimately, these reactions cause permanent damage to the cells.

Q: How do cytoprotective drugs counteract these chemical interactions?

A: Either by preventing the start of the cascade or by stopping its progression. According to a summary of recent research into the treatment of acute ischemic stroke, published in the July 21, 1993, *Journal of the American Medical Association,* the cytoprotective drugs now being tested include: calcium channel blockers, such as **nimodipine**, which could affect the buildup of calcium; drugs that block the channels of certain amino acids that encourage calcium accumulation; and free-radical scavengers, which could prevent cellular damage caused by oxygen free radicals—oxygen atoms that lack electrons. These scavengers include a group of drugs known as *lazaroids,* because their ability to restore brain function is comparable to Lazarus' resurrection from the dead (*Patient Care,* August 15, 1994). Also being tested are glutamate antagonists, which could prevent the cascade from starting.

INITIAL MEDICAL TREATMENT OF HEMORRHAGIC STROKE

Q: If any of these cytoprotective drugs come on the market, will they be used to treat hemorrhagic stroke?

A: They might. Both hemorrhagic and ischemic strokes ultimately result in ischemia, or oxygen deprivation, and it is ischemic brain cells that set off the glutamate cascade. But their use will depend upon whether or not they increase the risk of bleeding—and that has yet to be determined. Initial studies of these drugs are focusing primarily on their effectiveness in treating ischemic stroke, according to pharmaceutical researchers (*Drug*

Topics, April 19, 1993), although at least one free-radical scavenger, tirilazad mesylate, is being studied in sub-arachnoid hemorrhage (*Patient Care,* August 15, 1994).

Q: Then how do doctors treat hemorrhagic stroke?

A: The treatment of hemorrhagic stroke, like the treatment of ischemic stroke, depends on both the cause and the stage of the stroke. Generally speaking, however, doctors must stop the bleeding and reduce pressure on the brain. This is done with both medication and surgery.

Stopping Hemorrhage

Q: How do doctors stop bleeding from a hemorrhagic stroke?

A: In part, through medication. Controlling blood pressure is crucial. High blood pressure puts stress on the arteries and may contribute to or worsen hemorrhage. A reduction in blood pressure helps reduce that stress and may help stop bleeding. But, as in ischemic stroke, low blood pressure in hemorrhagic stroke can cause additional damage to the brain.

Q: I can see how controlling blood pressure could help control bleeding, but wouldn't the doctor have to actually close the ruptured vessel to stop the bleeding?

A: In many cases, yes. As we've just said, surgery is one of the methods for treating hemorrhagic stroke. The actual surgical procedure used, however, depends on the cause of the hemorrhage. If the stroke is caused by a ruptured blood vessel, the vessel can be surgically repaired; if it is caused by an aneurysm, the surgeon can surgically clip off the aneurysm and repair the vessel, removing any clots that have formed; and if it is caused by an arteriovenous malformation—a tangle of blood vessels in the brain—the malformation can be surgically removed.

Relieving Pressure

Q: Do any of these surgical procedures relieve the pressure on the brain caused by the escaped blood?

A: In and of themselves, no. But they do stop additional blood from leaking out and increasing the pressure. Another surgical procedure, known as **evacuation**, reduces the pressure. Evacuation, quite simply, is the draining of the pool of blood that accumulates in hemorrhagic stroke. This pool is known as a **hematoma**.

Q: When is evacuation performed?

A: Depending on a stroke victim's condition, evacuation may be the first line of treatment for hemorrhagic stroke. It is usually performed on an emergency basis when the pressure caused by a hematoma produces severe and life-threatening neurological dysfunction.

Q: Are any other emergency surgical procedures used to treat hemorrhagic stroke?

A: Yes, **ventriculostomy** is performed when a sub-arachnoid or cerebral hemorrhage bleeds into the brain's ventricles, small cavities filled with cerebrospinal fluid. Bleeding into these cavities can produce *hydrocephalus,* a potentially dangerous condition known as water on the brain. In ventriculostomy, an opening is created to allow the fluid and blood to drain.

Q: What if the hemorrhage began some time before the surgery and the blood has already begun to clot?

A: Surgical treatment for hemorrhagic stroke can also include clot removal.

Q: Are all hemorrhagic-stroke victims treated surgically?

A: No. The surgical treatment of stroke victims depends on their condition and the stage of their strokes. If performing surgery would place them at greater risk than allowing the stroke to continue its course, or if irreversible damage has already been done, surgery may not be an option or may be delayed. In these instances, they may be treated with medication and bed rest.

Q: What aspects of hemorrhagic stroke can medication treat?

A: Drugs are primarily used to reduce brain swelling, or **edema**, and prevent complications. Medications to reduce brain swelling include mannitol, a medication (composed of sugar) that reduces pressure in the brain, and diuretics.

To prevent **vasospasm**, an artery spasm that is common to subarachnoid hemorrhage and that can cause further brain damage, doctors may prescribe the calcium channel blocker nimodipine.

COMPLICATIONS OF STROKE

Q: So vasospasm is a complication of certain hemorrhagic strokes. Are there any other stroke complications I should be aware of?

A: Yes. Both hemorrhagic and ischemic stroke can produce a variety of complications, including brain swelling; seizures; **aspiration pneumonia**, which is an inflammatory condition of the lungs and bronchial tubes caused by taking foreign matter or vomit into the lungs; **pulmonary embolism**, a potentially life-threatening embolism in the lungs; cardiac abnormalities; depression; nutritional disorders; infection; bed sores and nerve compression. Prevention and treatment of these complications, along with efforts to prevent stroke recurrence, are the focus of the next phase of medical treatment.

Q: How are these complications treated?

A: Swelling is treated with diuretics or mannitol; seizures, with anticonvulsants; aspiration pneumonia, by suctioning the foreign material from the lungs and giving oxygen; and pulmonary embolism, with anticoagulants, such as heparin and warfarin and, in some cases, surgery. Pulmonary embolism, which is often caused by a clot in the vein of a leg affected by stroke, can also be prevented with low doses of anticoagulants or platelet inhibitors injected into the vein where the clot originated.

The treatment of cardiac abnormalities, discussed in Chapter 2, depends on the abnormality. Depression, which we discuss in more detail in Chapter 6, is treated with antidepressants and counseling. Nutritional disorders are treated with nutrition therapy and diet. Infection treatment varies according to its cause; generally, however, infections caused by bacteria are treated with antibiotics. Bed sores, which themselves can become infected, are discussed in Chapter 6.

POST-ACUTE-STROKE TREATMENT

Q: In addition to preventing and treating complications, you said the next phase of stroke treatment involves preventing recurrent stroke. How is this accomplished?

A: Again, the answer depends on the type of stroke. In hemorrhagic stroke, the next phase of treatment focuses on controlling risk factors, primarily hypertension. Because certain antihypertensive medications are inappropriate for hemorrhagic-stroke victims, the medications of choice are usually beta blockers and ACE inhibitors.

Other preventive treatments for victims of hemorrhagic stroke may include monitoring for hydrocephalus and, possibly, performing carotid endarterectomy.

In ischemic stroke, preventive treatment involves long-term therapy with either aspirin, ticlopidine or warfarin to prevent recurrent clot formation. It also involves monitoring and control of blood pressure and other risk factors; it may also include carotid endarterectomy.

In both types of stroke, post-acute treatment also includes rehabilitation, which is the topic of Chapter 6.

6 REHABILITATION

Q: What is the goal of rehabilitation?

A: Rehabilitation is designed to restore an individual to normal functioning (or as close to normal as possible) after a disease or injury. In stroke survivors, this can mean restoring functional as well as physical ability. For example, rehabilitation for a stroke survivor with hemiplegia may focus not only on restoring muscle function to the affected leg but also on using the leg's muscles—or other muscles—to get around. This could involve adaptation and compensation—perhaps a change in gait or the use of a cane, walker or wheelchair—as well as physical rehabilitation of the leg.

Q: But so many functions can be affected by stroke. Is any one health professional qualified to deal with them all?

A: Not really. It takes a team of medical and allied health professionals working with family members and friends to rehabilitate a stroke survivor.

Q: Who are the major players on this "team"?

A: Think of it as an "all-star team"—one in which each member plays a major role at some point. First at bat are the medical experts—the doctors and nurses who handle the medical crisis, prepare the stroke survivor for rehabilitation and monitor his health during the rehabilitation process. In time, assorted therapists and counselors take the plate, helping the survivor regain functional ability and strength and come to grips with the changes caused by his stroke. Batting cleanup are the family members and friends who help the professionals and provide needed love and support.

At any given point during the rehabilitation process, any one of these players could be considered the star. But perhaps the real star of the team is the stroke survivor— the only player who never gets a chance to sit on the bench and rest. The survivor is as much or more a part of the rehabilitation team as the professionals—his overall attitude and his attitude toward rehabilitation have a major effect on its success.

Q: I can see how the survivor's attitude would be important. But success must also depend on the other team members. Can we discuss these players in more detail?

A: Certainly. We've already learned much about the role of the doctor, but we haven't yet looked at her training or that of her colleagues. Depending on the severity of the stroke, the age of the survivor and where he receives his emergency treatment, several doctors may be assigned to the team. The team could include the survivor's personal physician—an internist or general or family practitioner—as well as specialists, such as **neurologists, physiatrists, geriatricians,** and perhaps **cardiologists, neurosurgeons** or **urologists.**

All of these professionals are physicians—they've completed medical school and received their M.D. or D.O. degrees. All of the specialists, and perhaps even the survivor's primary-care doctor, have also completed at least three years of specialty training known as a residency. In addition, some may also have completed additional training in a subspecialty.

Q: **Can you tell me a little bit more about the specialists? For instance, what does a neurologist do?**

A: A neurologist specializes in the diagnosis and treatment of problems involving the nervous system—the brain, spinal cord, motor and sensory nerves, muscles and involuntary nervous system—and the related blood vessels. It is often the neurologist who takes charge of the initial diagnosis and treatment of stroke. During rehabilitation, he may serve either as the primary doctor or as a consultant.

Q: **What is a physiatrist?**

A: A physiatrist is a doctor who specializes in physical medicine and rehabilitation. He diagnoses, evaluates and treats people with disabilities or impairments involving the musculoskeletal, neurologic and cardio-vascular systems. His primary focus is on restoring function and alleviating pain. As you might guess, he may play a major role in the rehabilitation process.

Q: What role might a geriatrician play in rehabilitating a stroke survivor?

A: Remember, stroke becomes more common as a person ages. Many stroke survivors are elderly and must deal with other problems of aging in addition to their strokes. A geriatrician—a family practice doctor or internist who subspecializes in the care of older people—can deal with those problems as well as the effects of stroke.

Q: What about the other specialists? Am I right in assuming their participation on the rehabilitation team depends on the survivor's situation?

A: You certainly are. A cardiologist, or heart specialist, would be part of the team if the survivor has heart problems or if his stroke was cardiac in origin. A neurosurgeon, a surgeon who specializes in the nervous system, would be called upon if surgery were necessary, although she is also qualified to diagnose, evaluate, treat and rehabilitate stroke survivors. And a urologist would likely join the team if the survivor developed a urinary-tract infection or continence problem.

Q: Which doctor is actually responsible for the survivor's primary care?

A: That depends. In some instances, the survivor's primary-care physician heads the medical team. In others, a neurologist or physiatrist serves as captain, coordinating care with the other doctors, nurses and, if nutritional problems are involved, a dietitian or nutritionist.

Q: **Didn't you say that the rehabilitation team might also include therapists?**

A: Yes. Depending on the effects of the stroke, a survivor may need the services of a **physical therapist**, an **occupational therapist**, a **speech therapist** (also called a **speech-language pathologist**) or a **recreational therapist**. These therapists, respectively, help the stroke survivor regain the use of his limbs, independence, communication skills and social skills. We'll discuss the roles of these allied health professionals in more detail when we examine the therapies they offer.

Q: **Are there any other members of the rehabilitation team?**

A: Yes. Remember, stroke produces psychological effects in addition to physical and cognitive ones. An estimated 30 to 60 percent of stroke survivors suffer from depression, and the vast majority of stroke survivors —and their families—require some help adjusting to stroke's effects. Because of this, the stroke team may also include a psychiatrist, a psychologist, one or more social workers and a vocational counselor.

Both the psychiatrist and the psychologist can treat depression; in addition, they and various social workers can help the stroke survivor—and her family—adjust to the new circumstances. Social workers may also be instrumental in helping the family prepare for the survivor's return home. And a vocational counselor can help the survivor choose and train for a new career if the effects of her stroke have made her unable to return to her old one.

Q: I hadn't thought that far ahead. I guess rehabilitation is more involved than I thought. How long does it take?

A: That depends. Some stroke survivors need little or no rehabilitation—perhaps only days or weeks; others are so severely injured that they do not benefit much from any amount of rehabilitation. For those in the middle, the process can last weeks, months or years. The bulk of the recovery, however, usually comes during the first year after the stroke.

Q: Does the survivor stay in the hospital the whole time?

A: Generally, no. Rehabilitation usually begins in the hospital, then continues after discharge—either in a **rehabilitation center** or at home.

Q: What is a rehabilitation center?

A: A rehabilitation center is a specialized institution that provides professional rehabilitation services—physical, occupational and speech therapy, nursing, social services, psychology and perhaps vocational counseling—to disabled persons to help them attain their maximum functional capacity. These centers, which may or may not be affiliated with a hospital, usually provide services on both an outpatient and inpatient basis.

Q: How can I find a rehabilitation center?

A: Rehabilitation centers are located in most large communities. Depending on where you live, there may be several in your community. You can begin your search for a center by asking your doctor and the hospital staff for their recommendations. Then learn as much as you can about the facilities they've recommended.

Check to see if the facilities are licensed and accredited. Licensing requirements vary from state to state, but accreditation is done on a national basis by both the Commission on the Accreditation of Rehabilitation Facilities and the Joint Commission on the Accreditation of Healthcare Organizations. Accreditation by either commission means that the facility meets certain standards. (For more information, see the section "Informational and Mutual-Aid Groups" at the back of the book.)

Find out what services the facilities offer, what equipment is available and how accessible the facilities are. Ask about the qualifications of the staff members—are they licensed or certified? Do they work together as a team? Ask what they will do to help the stroke survivor prepare for his return home—will they visit and assess your home and help you line up needed equipment and services? Finally, ask whether the facilities accept the patient's insurance and whether his insurance will cover the rehabilitation services he needs.

Q: Can we backtrack a bit? We're choosing a rehabilitation center before the rehabilitation process has started. Didn't you say rehabilitation usually begins in the hospital?

A: Yes. In fact, rehabilitation often starts soon after the medical emergency is over, as various team members assess the damage caused by the stroke and begin to work with the survivor. In these early stages, their work may not require the survivor's active participation. It may involve positioning him to prevent bedsores and damage to his muscles and joints, or it may mean moving his arms and legs to retain the joints' **range of motion**, or ability to move.

As the stroke survivor becomes more alert and regains some strength, concentration and control, however, he will assume his place on the team and begin working toward a prescribed set of goals—goals that may include relearning old motor skills, learning how to adapt and compensate for various impairments, mastering activities of daily living, regaining communication skills, and coping with stroke and the changes it has caused.

Q: Are these goals worked toward simultaneously?

A: If you mean are they worked toward over the same period of time, the answer is yes. The rehabilitation team does not focus on one problem at a time—it does not, for example, wait until physical abilities are restored before addressing communication problems. At any given moment, the stroke survivor may be working toward a variety of goals.

PHYSICAL REHABILITATION

Q: Can we break the rehabilitation process into its various types and look at each in more detail, beginning with physical rehabilitation?

A: Certainly. As we mentioned above, physical rehabilitation can begin soon after the stroke emergency ends. Positioning, for example, often begins even before the stroke survivor regains consciousness.

Passive Stage

Q: Why is that?

A: When people are bed- or chair-ridden for long periods of time, the lack of movement places continuous pressure on the skin that covers bony areas, such as the hips and shoulders. This persistent pressure can impede blood flow and kill tissue, resulting in **decubitus ulcers**, or bedsores. These sores, which are treated by cleaning the area and applying topical medications, take a long time to heal and can be life-threatening if they become infected. So the rehabilitation team's goal is to prevent them. In people who can move—even slightly—bedsores can be prevented by shifting weight periodically or by moving, stretching, rolling or turning over. A stroke survivor who is unconscious or paralyzed, however, cannot do this. So members of the rehabilitation team, often nurses, must move his body for him to prevent the buildup of pressure.

Positioning also helps prevent joint damage. When a person loses feeling and control of the muscles in a leg or arm, that leg or arm may position itself unnaturally. In a bedridden person, for example, the leg may turn out from the hip. This can damage the hip joint and prevent the leg from regaining normal function. The rehabilitation team must position the leg properly to prevent this damage.

Q: Can the rehabilitation team do anything else before the stroke survivor is able to participate actively?

A: Yes. You probably know from experience that inactivity of certain muscles and joints can affect their flexibility. If you haven't done a split for 20 years, for example, chances are you won't be able to do one now. Since you probably have little need to perform such gymnastics, this is unlikely to present a problem. In a stroke survivor, however, inactivity may affect more commonly used muscles and joints. And, as the saying goes, a person who doesn't move it can lose it.

To prevent this from happening, the rehabilitation team moves the affected limbs within their range of motion—the extent to which the various joints can move. These range-of-motion exercises help maintain the flexibility of the joints and muscles.

Q: **Which member of the rehabilitation team performs these exercises?**

A: The primary "exerciser" is the physical therapist.

Q: **What exactly does a physical therapist do?**

A: The physical therapist is an allied health professional who is licensed to assist in testing and treating physically disabled people. She uses exercise, massage, movement, heat, light, sound waves and other therapies to help restore functional movement, prevent disability and pain, and promote healing.

Active Stage

Q: Which therapy does the physical therapist use when the stroke survivor is ready to participate actively in rehabilitation?

A: That depends on the extent and stage of paralysis. In general, however, the physical therapist or a physiatrist will test the survivor to learn what she can and cannot do, then develop a rehabilitation plan that establishes step-by-step goals. A common rehabilitation plan would have bed mobility as its first goal, followed by sitting, standing and, finally, walking.

Q: You just used the phrase "stage of paralysis." Are there different ones?

A: Yes. The first is **flaccidity**. In this stage, both muscle tone and reflexive and voluntary movement are absent. The affected limb is limp and floppy. The flaccid stage is usually followed by **beginning spasticity**, in which muscle tone begins to return, along with some reflexive, or involuntary, movement. Beginning spasticity is followed by **full spasticity**, in which the muscles have excessive tone, reflexes are hyperactive and there is little control of voluntary movement. At this stage, the muscles are abnormally stiff and resistent to stretching, and there is a danger of developing **contractures**— shortened, tightened tissues around a joint. These contractures prevent muscles from lengthening, immobilize the joint and reduce the range of motion.

The final stage of paralysis occurs when the muscles begin to approach normal tone. In this stage, **spasticity** decreases and voluntary movement increases. It's important to note, however, that these stages may overlap or be skipped altogether.

Q: What kind of physical rehabilitation is appropriate to each stage?

A: Range-of-motion exercises and proper positioning are the keystones of rehabilitation in the flaccid stage. Splints may be added when spasticity begins, in order to better control positioning. By the time a survivor reaches the full-spasticity stage, rehabilitation includes added sets of range-of-motion and stretching exercises, in which he actually participates. And when his muscles approach normal tone, rehabilitation will also include relaxation and strengthening exercises.

Exercise

Q: Physical therapy seems to include a lot of exercise. Why is that?

A: There are several reasons. Exercise enables a survivor to maintain and perhaps increase his freedom of movement; it stretches tight muscles and helps relax spasticity and prevent contractures, so that the muscles can be trained to operate properly again; and it increases strength in limbs weakened by stroke. In addition, exercise helps improve circulation and decrease the swelling common to a stroke survivor's inactive body parts.

Positioning Devices and Other Therapies

Q:
You mentioned splints. Do they help with exercise?

A:
Not directly. Splints and other devices simply keep the muscles and joints in proper position and prevent damage and contractures. A common sling, for example, can be used to hold a flaccid arm close to the body to prevent it from hanging like a dead weight and causing **subluxation**, or partial dislocation, of the shoulder joint. A hand splint or a cone held in the hand can be used during the spastic stage to keep the affected hand in a functional position, with fingers open, thumb curving from the palm and the wrist slightly extended. Braces may be used to keep a leg from turning out or to support a weak ankle, and lap boards and arm troughs—devices that attach to wheelchairs—can provide support for an affected arm when seated.

Q:
Does physical therapy include anything other than exercise?

A:
It can. Physical therapists and physiatrists may use a variety of other therapies, including water, heat, light, electricity and ultrasound, to stimulate or relax muscles.

• Whirlpool baths can ease muscle-spasm pain.

• Heat—applied through hot-water compresses, infrared lamps, shortwave radiation, electrical current, ultrasound or warm baths—can be used to stimulate circulation and relax tense muscles.

• Low-intensity electrical currents can be applied through the skin to stimulate weak muscles and make them contract.

Walking

Q: When does a survivor actually begin walking?

A: That depends on several things: her body's ability to heal, the severity of the problem, her attitude, when rehabilitation began (the sooner, the better) and the aggressiveness of therapy. Generally speaking, however, walking becomes possible when the survivor has enough strength in at least one leg and her trunk to compensate for her weakness, when her unaffected arm is capable of holding and bearing down on a cane or walker, and when she has regained some sense of balance. Before she learns to walk, however, she must first learn to sit up and to stand.

During this same time, she may also learn how to **transfer** from her bed to a wheelchair and from her wheelchair to the toilet, and learn how to move her wheelchair independently. These skills enable her to regain independence while she remasters the art of walking.

Q: Do most stroke survivors regain the ability to walk?

A: The majority do, although many require walking aids.

Q: What kind of walking aids are available?

A: There are a variety of walking aids available, and many survivors progress from one to another over the course of rehabilitation. They may take their first steps with the aid of parallel bars, for example, then progress to a hemi-walker (a combination cane and walker for one-sided use) or large-based quad-cane (a cane with four legs to provide added support). From a large-based quad-cane, they may move to a quad-cane with a small base or to a standard cane. Eventually, they may be able to walk without any walking aid.

Q: What about the arm and hand? Do their functions return at the same time as the leg?

A: In general, restoration of arm and hand function follows that of the leg. The leg, with its larger muscles, simply responds better to rehabilitation than the arm, which has smaller, more delicate muscles. And the hand, whose muscles are smaller still, usually responds only after function has returned to the arm. In many cases, a stroke survivor will regain full use of her affected leg but not the affected arm.

OCCUPATIONAL THERAPY

Q: Can anything be done to help those who don't regain the full use of their arms or hands?

A: Yes. In fact, that is often a major part of occupational therapy. The occupational therapist's job is to help stroke survivors master the activities of daily living and become more independent. Since many of these activities normally involve the use of both hands, the occupational therapist may have to teach alternative methods. In fact, teaching and training, as well as practice and exercise, are key methods used by these allied health professionals.

Q: When does occupational therapy begin?

A: Generally, it begins in the hospital, as soon as a survivor is able to actively participate. Think about it: Stroke's effects can prevent a person from controlling her bladder and bowels, from bathing, eating, drinking, dressing and taking care of herself—activities she's taken for granted for years. The loss of these abilities can be very degrading to a survivor, so the sooner they are regained, the better the person feels. Remastering these once-simple tasks can not only boost self-esteem, but also can give the survivor hope that she can overcome stroke's other effects.

Q: Which activities are tackled first?

A: The occupational therapist may begin by teaching the bedridden survivor to roll over or prop herself up, using the unaffected part of her body. He may teach her how to use a bedpan and, ultimately, how to maneuver in the bathroom. If the stroke has affected the survivor's stronger hand, the occupational therapist may have to teach her how to wash or feed herself with her weaker hand. Even if the weaker hand was affected by the stroke, the survivor may need help performing these tasks with only one hand. But beyond feeding, eating itself can be a problem if the survivor has difficulty swallowing.

Swallowing

Q: How does the therapist know if there's a swallowing problem?

A: If a person coughs or chokes when she eats, or feels like food is getting stuck in her throat, she may have a swallowing disorder. To determine this for certain, one or more members of the team—usually the occupational therapist, speech therapist, nutritionist or doctor—performs a swallowing evaluation—watching as the survivor chews and swallows. If this evaluation does not produce results, the team may order a **barium swallow**. In this test, the survivor swallows barium sulfate then undergoes a series of x-rays. The barium shows up on the x-rays, illustrating both the swallowing process and the gastrointestinal tract. The team can then detect any problems involved.

Q: How are swallowing problems treated?

A: In most stroke survivors, swallowing therapy— special exercises for coordinating the swallowing muscles or restimulating the nerves that trigger the swallowing reflex—can take care of the problem. Swallowing therapy is usually provided by a speech therapist or occupational therapist. One of them can also teach a survivor how to place food in her mouth or how to position her body and head to help facilitate swallowing.

Eating

Q: Are there any other ways that an occupational therapist can help a survivor learn to eat?

A: Poor posture, weakness in half of the mouth, inadequate lip closure and visual and perceptual problems, such as hemianopia or one-sided neglect, can all affect a person's ability to eat. The occupational therapist can improve the survivor's posture, perhaps by changing or adjusting her chair. He can help her strengthen her mouth and lip muscles, and he can turn her plate or remind her where to look for the rest of her meal. He can work with a nutritionist or dietitian to make sure she is getting the proper nutrients in her diet in a form that she can swallow. And he can teach her to use adaptive equipment to make eating easier.

Q: What type of adaptive equipment is available?

A: Numerous items are available to enable a stroke survivor to eat independently. Plate guards, which add a metal rim to the outer edge of a plate, enable a person with one usable hand to scoop up food; double-sided sticky material can help anchor the plate in place. Rocker knives allow a person to cut food with only one hand; and built-up handles allow a person with little hand strength to hold and use utensils. Additionally, there are swivel spoons, which counteract wrist problems. These items are available through supply and catalog companies. Check with an occupational therapist, or refer to the section "Sources for Adaptive Clothing and Equipment" for purchasing information.

Continence Training

Q: **Are there any other activities of daily living that the occupational therapist can tackle early in the rehabilitation process?**

A: Yes. If the survivor has continence problems, the occupational therapist may provide bowel or bladder retraining.

Q: **What is that?**

A: Basically, it's an adult version of toilet training. It generally involves teaching the survivor to identify the urge to urinate or defecate and signal for assistance when the urge is felt. It may also involve establishing a pattern or schedule. For example, a person might visit the bathroom or be given a bedpan every two hours whether he has to use it or not. This provides him with an opportunity to go before it becomes necessary. It also helps prevent accidents.

Dressing

Q: **What else does occupational therapy include?**

A: Dressing is another major goal of occupational therapy. The ability to dress oneself can make a survivor feel more self-sufficient, and the idea of wearing street clothes instead of hospital gowns or pajamas can be emotionally uplifting. Training in dressing usually begins when the survivor is able to sit up.

Dressing can be a difficult process when half of the body doesn't cooperate. A stroke survivor is usually taught to put his clothing on his affected limbs first. In undressing, however, he should start with the unaffected limbs. It may take some time for the survivor to master this skill completely.

Q: What should the stroke survivor wear?

A: In general, the therapist will have the survivor dress in comfortable clothes that are easy to get on and fasten—e.g., slacks or skirts with elastic waistbands; loose-fitting, pullover tops; and clothing that fastens in the front. He may suggest that clothing be adapted to fasten with Velcro or snaps, or that Velcro- or snap-fastening clothing be purchased.

Q: What happens after these skills are recovered? Is that the end of occupational therapy?

A: Not necessarily. The occupational therapist may work to fine-tune or upgrade the patient's skills as abilities are regained. If, for example, control of his hand returns, the survivor may learn to use a regular knife, rather than a rocker knife. For some patients, the therapist may need to teach additional coping skills and methods of adapting if it becomes apparent that the arm or hand will not recover fully. The survivor may need to learn about the types of adaptive equipment available and how to use them. And once the survivor returns home, the occupational therapist can help with a number of other daily tasks that most people take for granted.

Q: So occupational therapy can continue at home?

A: Yes. So can physical therapy, speech therapy and other forms of rehabilitation. As we said earlier, rehabilitation usually begins in the hospital, then continues at a rehabilitation center or at home. If the rehabilitation team believes progress can continue after discharge, the doctor prescribes additional therapy, which can be obtained on either an outpatient basis or at home. We'll discuss where to find home services in the next chapter.

SPEECH THERAPY

Q: Can you tell me more about speech therapy?

A: Certainly. Speech therapy—or more accurately, communication therapy—is provided by a speech-language pathologist—a nonmedical professional who holds a graduate degree in speech-language pathology. It involves the measurement and evaluation of both language abilities and speech production, and makes use of non-medical therapies to treat communication disorders, including problems in speaking, writing, reading and understanding verbal communication.

Q: When does speech therapy begin and what does it involve?

A: Like other forms of therapy, speech therapy generally begins as soon as possible. The actual form it takes depends on the actual language problem caused by the stroke. To determine the problem and its extent, the speech pathologist usually starts by administering assessment tests.

Q: What exactly is tested?

A: Primarily, speaking and listening. To determine language ability, for example, the speech pathologist may simply engage the survivor in conversation. While he is talking, she will monitor how much he speaks, how easily he speaks, the length and type of his sentences, and the amount of information he conveys. After she speaks, she will monitor how he responds to and understands words, sentences and paragraphs. She may test his ability to name objects, imitate words or sounds, read aloud and understand what he reads. She may ask him to write, draw or do arithmetic—all skills that deal with expressive communication. And she will monitor his ability to communicate through gesture. This can give her an idea which language abilities are intact and which have been affected by the stroke. Once she has determined the cause of the problem, therapy can begin.

Q: What does the actual therapy involve?

A: That depends on the type of problem and its cause. As you know, there are numerous communication problems associated with stroke. Here's an example.

Let's say the survivor has a speaking problem caused by an inability to control his speech muscles. The speech pathologist may begin by exercising and retraining those muscles. Once the muscles are functioning properly, she will help the survivor use them to produce sounds and, ultimately, words. She may, for example, explain how the sounds are made, manipulate the survivor's face and give him cues as to where his tongue should be or how his mouth should be positioned when he is saying the words. Eventually, they will progress to sentences, paragraphs and, finally, improved speaking capability.

Q: How does the survivor communicate in the meantime?

A: That depends on his deficit. Generally, the speech pathologist, who has learned the survivor's communication strengths through testing, encourages him to use those strengths to communicate in the best way he can. If he cannot speak but can write, for example, she will encourage him to write or use gestures to communicate. The goal of speech therapy is not only to restore as much speech or language capability as possible, but also to teach the survivor how to compensate for lost functions. This is important, because not every survivor with a speech or language deficit regains his full communication abilities. Most do, however, regain at least some of their abilities. And the speech pathologist can help family members and friends learn to better communicate with those with lasting deficits.

Q: How? Are there any general rules to follow?

A: Yes. First, remember what was affected—the survivor's language abilities, not his intellectual abilities. He may be dumb but he is not stupid. Don't talk down to him, don't insult him, and don't shout at him. He is not deaf. He may understand what you are saying but cannot respond.

If he has difficulty understanding, try to make it easier for him. Here are some suggestions:

- Get his attention before you speak to him.

- Slow down your speech.

- Use short, simple sentences and communicate one idea at a time.

- Give him time to process what you've said.

- If he doesn't understand, find another way to say what you mean.

- Use gestures, pictures or writing, if that makes comprehension easier.

And finally, be understanding. Realize that communication is hard work for him, and that his efforts may be both frustrating and tiring.

COUNSELING

Q: **How does a rehabilitation team help survivors cope with the frustration caused by communication problems and other effects of stroke?**

A: Primarily through counseling. Mental-health professionals counsel stroke survivors individually, with their families or in a group to help them come to grips with stroke's effects. Family and friends play a major role, offering needed love and support.

Q: **Other than frustration, what emotional reactions are common to stroke survivors?**

A: Immediate reactions often include disappointment, anger and fear. Later, some survivors enter a stage of denial or disbelief, in which they underestimate the degree of their impairment. Eventually, they begin to accept reality. At this point, many survivors go into a state of mourning for the loss of their abilities and former lifestyles—and many become depressed.

Q: **Is there any way to tell if a stroke survivor is depressed?**

A: Several physical and psychological clues may indicate depression in a stroke survivor. If she loses her appetite, loses weight, lacks energy, seems fatigued or has difficulty sleeping; if she seems to show little interest in herself, others or rehabilitation; or if she is pessimistic or exhibits low self-esteem, she may be depressed.

Q: **I know we've touched on this before, but how is depression treated?**

A: Depression can be treated with psychotherapy (counseling) or antidepressant drugs. The member of the rehabilitation team who handles this treatment is usually a psychiatrist, psychologist or clinical social worker. Treatment, which can take place in a hospital or rehabilitation center, can also be done on an outpatient basis after the stroke survivor returns home. But it should begin as soon as possible after depression is diagnosed, because depression can have a negative impact on rehabilitation.

Q: What other roles do these mental-health professionals play in rehabilitating stroke survivors?

A: Generally, they counsel survivors—and their families—about how to accept and cope with the changes caused by stroke. Think about it: Stroke alters self-image and reminds people of their mortality and vulnerability. It causes physical and mental changes, affects relationships, and can greatly alter people's social lives. Stroke survivors—and their families—need to discuss and react to these changes. They need to learn how these changes will affect their future lives, and what methods they can use to cope. This can be accomplished through individual, family or group counseling, as well as through participation in support groups.

Q: At what stage during the rehabilitation process does counseling take place?

A: Counseling can occur during any part of the rehabilitation process. It may begin in the hospital or the rehabilitation center and follow the stroke survivor home, or it may begin at home, as the survivor and her family come to grips with their changing relationships.

Q: How does stroke affect a person's relationships?

A: Quite definitively. It can place a parent in the role of a child; or a child, spouse or sibling can take the role of parent. A vibrant, independent person can suddenly become dependent on her family members; the family members, in turn, who may be unaccustomed to having someone depend on them, can suddenly find themselves overcome with new responsibilities. A stay-at-home spouse may suddenly have to get a job to support the family; adult children may suddenly have to juggle caring for their parent with caring for their own children; and siblings may suddenly find themselves intimately involved in the lives of family members they haven't lived with for years. These changes are difficult for everyone involved to accept. And to top it off, the survivor and her family members may also have to deal with unexpected personality changes.

Q: **No wonder both the survivor and the family need counseling. Didn't you say this can affect their social lives, too?**

A: Yes. Both the survivor and her family may see a noticeable decrease in social life. During the first few months, both may be so caught up in rehabilitation and adjustment that they have little time for socializing. If the stroke has affected the survivor physically, she may be unable to go out, get around and socialize; if it has affected her communication skills, she may be unable to speak and socialize. She may feel self-conscious about her capabilities, be depressed or feel isolated. In addition, her emotional state and changes in her mental functions and personality can affect her social life.

But the survivor and her family are not the only ones who may withdraw. Friends who don't understand stroke and its effects—including the personality changes and the weight of responsibilities assumed by family members— may be uncomfortable and stop visiting.

Q: **Can the counseling team address these problems?**

A: Yes. And so, to some extent, can the survivor's family. The family can make a concerted effort to include the survivor in activities and offer emotional support and encouragement. They can briefly explain stroke and its effects to the survivor's friends, and they can make sure they make some time for themselves—time to meet their own social needs.

Q: Is there anything else that can be done to help a withdrawn stroke survivor?

A: A withdrawn stroke survivor might benefit from recreational therapy, which uses games or other group actions to spark social interests or make speaking to others easier. These activities, often planned and coordinated by a recreational therapist, are offered at many rehabilitation centers.

Recreational therapy can also be used to enhance the cognitive skills affected by stroke. A therapist might ask a person with planning and organizing deficits to play chess or checkers, or have a survivor with perceptual skills play Scrabble or bingo, or do word searches, crossword puzzles or jigsaw puzzles.

Q: Rehabilitation itself seems to be a giant puzzle, with each team member providing her own important piece. But I want to know how all the pieces fit together. What is a typical day like?

A: That depends on the stage of rehabilitation and where it's taking place. In the early stages, at the hospital, the primary focus is on the stroke survivor's health. Short sessions of therapy may be interspersed with medical care and bed rest throughout the day. As the survivor improves, therapy sessions increase in length, and the amount of medical care needed decreases.

Gradually, rehabilitation becomes the primary focus. During this intensive phase, the stroke survivor's day is filled from morning till night with activities related to rehabilitation. During a typical day in a rehabilitation center, for example, the survivor gets up, washes and gets dressed—activities that involve practicing newly learned or relearned skills. He then eats breakfast—again practicing skills—before starting a series of therapy sessions. After lunch, he may take a short nap, then have several more therapy sessions before dinner. In the evenings, he may visit with family, do exercises prescribed by his various therapists and, possibly, participate in recreational therapy before getting ready for bed—again practicing newly learned or relearned skills.

Q: **How long does this type of schedule go on?**

A: Until the members of the rehabilitation team feel that the survivor is either ready to go home or has been rehabilitated to the best of his ability.

Neither instance necessarily means that the survivor is ready to resume his normal lifestyle. The first may mean that the survivor's need for medical care and constant professional attention has decreased enough that he can continue his rehabilitation at home, where his day may be a little less structured but still full of therapy, exercise and practice. The second may mean that no further progress can be made. In the latter case, depending on the survivor's condition and the situation at his home, the team may recommend that the survivor move into a nursing home or some other type of assisted living arrangement. We'll discuss the factors that figure into this decision in the next chapter.

7 HOME AGAIN

Q: **Who determines where a stroke survivor will go after he is discharged from the hospital or rehabilitation center?**

A: Depending on the individual situation, any or all members of the rehabilitation team may play a part in deciding what place the stroke survivor will call "home."

When most stroke survivors think of going home, they think about returning to the homes in which they lived before they had their strokes. In many cases, those are the homes to which they return. But if they lived alone or lived with a person who is not capable of providing the care they need—perhaps someone with health problems of her own—home may become the house of a relative or friend or a nursing home or some other type of assisted-living facility. These facilities can also become home to stroke survivors who require more medical or personal care than they can receive safely, efficiently and cost-effectively in a private home.

Q: What types of assisted-living arrangements are there?

A: Three major types of facilities are available. At the top of the list are **skilled nursing facilities**, which offer nursing services similar to those given in a hospital. There are also **intermediate-care facilities**, which provide less-intensive care than skilled nursing facilities, and **residential care homes**, which offer what is known as **custodial care** (room, board and personal services). Some facilities offer all three types of care.

Q: What determines whether a stroke survivor will need to move into one of these facilities or whether he will be able to return to a private home?

A: A number of factors go into this decision, including the survivor's physical and emotional strengths and weaknesses. In other words, the rehabilitation team looks at how many activities of daily living he can perform, his ability to communicate, his medical problems, the number of medications he needs, the amount of professional services he needs and his emotional state.

In addition, the team must consider his home environment—whether a family member or friend is available to serve as a caregiver; whether that caregiver is healthy and strong; what the social and economic needs of the family are; how the family feels about the survivor's return; what financial resources are available; whether insurance will cover home care; whether financial assistance is available to cover home care; whether the necessary support services are available and whether the physical layout of the house is suitable.

PREPARING THE HOME

Q: What type of private home is most appropriate for a stroke survivor?

A: That depends on the survivor's limitations and capabilities. A survivor who is wheelchair-bound, for example, needs a home that is wheelchair-accessible. So does a survivor who is mastering the art of walking but who still relies on a wheelchair to get around. Even a survivor who has no need for a wheelchair may have trouble with stairs, bathrooms, kitchens and other setups we often take for granted. Generally speaking, however, ranch houses and houses that have amenities, including bathrooms, on the first floor, are most appropriate. But adaptation can make living in other types of houses feasible as well.

Q: Let's say the survivor lives with me. Can anyone help me determine if my home fits the bill?

A: Yes. In fact, the hospital or rehabilitation center generally assigns a social worker or other staff member to visit the home of a stroke survivor who is about to be discharged to assess its accessibility and determine what, if any, adjustments should be made before he comes home.

Q: What specific things will the social worker look for?

A: Taking into consideration the abilities and limitations of the stroke survivor, the social worker will look at the walkways, entrances, doorways and halls, as well as the physical layout and furnishings of the home. If the survivor is wheelchair-bound, for example, doorways and hallways must be measured to determine whether the wheelchair can fit through. A ground-floor bathroom is also a major consideration. And if the survivor walks with the aid of a quad-cane, stair steps must be long enough and wide enough to accommodate the cane.

Depending on the social worker's findings, a number of changes may be recommended to make the house accessible: Perhaps an entrance ramp should be built, or a rear or side entrance should become the primary entrance for the stroke survivor; or perhaps a first-floor room will need to be transformed into a bedroom.

Q: What other changes might be recommended?

A: Both wheelchair-bound survivors and survivors who are still mastering walking skills need smooth surfaces to ride or walk on and as few obstacles as possible. With that in mind, plush, deep-pile carpeting, loose scatter rugs or cracked walkways may need to be replaced; electrical cords may need to be secured or moved; furniture may need to be rearranged to allow greater maneuverability; and areas the survivor will use will need to be well lit.

Steps should be marked with colored or reflective tape to make them easier to see; railings should be installed in all stairways used by the stroke survivor; and cushions or pillows may need to be placed on chairs and sofas to raise the level of the seats—to make it easier for the survivor to stand up and sit down.

In the bathroom, nonslip pads, mats or decals may need to be put in the tub or shower and grab bars may need to be installed. A bath or shower seat and a shower hose may be suggested to facilitate bathing. If there is no bathroom on the first floor, a commode chair can be used temporarily.

Major renovation recommendations for the wheelchair-bound could include widening doors; building ramps; lowering counters, light switches and thermostats; and installing a roll-in shower and higher toilet in the bathroom and an elevator lift to the second floor. Because these renovations are costly and take some time to complete, the social worker may suggest that the survivor look for other living arrangements, at least temporarily.

Q: You mentioned a commode chair. Where could I get something like that?

A: Numerous companies sell and lease durable medical equipment, such as commode chairs, hospital beds and wheelchairs. The social worker or someone else on the hospital or rehabilitation-center staff can help you determine which types of equipment may be useful for you and whether you should buy or rent. He can also provide you with names of suppliers in your area.

Q: What else must be done before my family member comes home?

A: In addition to preparing your house and lining up necessary equipment, you'll need to know what services the survivor will need and where they will come from. In other words, you need a **discharge plan**, or **management plan**. This plan, developed by the rehabilitation team, outlines the survivor's medical and therapy needs, and establishes how rehabilitation and daily care will continue once the survivor is discharged from the hospital or rehabilitation center.

DETERMINING NEEDS

Q:

What does this plan include?

A:

That depends on both the survivor's situation and that of the rehabilitation team. Medically, it might include a list of the medications the survivor is supposed to take; information about what, if any, continuing nursing care is needed; instructions about the frequency and location of medical exams and monitoring; instructions about lifestyle changes to prevent stroke; and prescriptions for additional therapy.

Details of the plan might stipulate how often physical, occupational or speech therapy will continue, who will conduct it and where it will take place. The survivor's personal needs will also be addressed. If she needs help dressing or bathing, for example, the plan will identify those needs and address how they will be met. It might, for example, suggest that a **personal-care aide** be added to the rehabilitation team after the survivor is discharged or that family members be trained to assume these caregiving roles.

Q:

Do family members have a say in this?

A:

They certainly do. After all, the family is an important part of the rehabilitation team, and the lives of its members are greatly affected by their loved one's return. They should help determine their own roles in the continuing rehabilitation of the survivor, as well as where rehabilitation will take place. If, for example, they are able to transport the survivor to an outpatient center on a regular basis, outpatient rehabilitation may be included in the discharge plan. If they cannot provide transportation, the plan may stipulate that therapists and other members of the rehabilitation team provide services in the home.

LINING UP HOME SERVICES

Q: What types of home services are available?

A: A multitude of services are available for the stroke survivor and her family—from medical care and therapy, to the proverbial soup to nuts (meal services). These services, provided by **home health agencies**, private companies, service organizations and volunteers, include medical care; nursing care; physical, occupational and speech therapy; the services of **home health aides** and personal-care aides; housekeeping; meal services and adult day care. For the family members or caregivers, there is **respite care**, to give the primary caregivers a needed break. And for stroke survivors who are functional and independent enough to live alone, there are **checking services** that check in every now and then to see if things are going well.

Q: Can we take a closer look at some of these services?

A: Certainly. Let's take them in order. Both medical and nursing care can be provided in the home. You may or may not remember the old-fashioned house call. Although rare, it does still exist, but its existence depends on the doctor. It may also depend on the mobility of the stroke patient. Some doctors who do not generally make house calls may make exceptions for patients who cannot come to their offices.

Nurses, too, make house calls. In fact, visiting nurses are generally the keystone of most home-health agencies. Both registered and practical nurses offer services in the home, including dressing wounds, changing catheters, monitoring vital signs and overall health status, administering medications, giving injections, monitoring special dietary regimens and instructing family members or other nonprofessional caregivers. They can provide round-the-clock services if needed, or pay regularly scheduled visits.

Q: How can I find home nursing care?

A: Start by asking the members of the rehabilitation team. They may be able to recommend a home health agency that provides the nursing services you need. These agencies, which can be privately owned, hospital-based or, like the Visiting Nurse Associations of America, nonprofit in nature, employ nurses who work solely in the patients' homes.

Usually listed in the yellow pages of the phone book under the heading "home health care," home health agencies may also be able to put you in touch with physical, occupational and speech therapists who offer therapy sessions in the home, and home health aides and personal-care aides who can provide an assortment of helpful services.

Q: What should I look for in choosing a home health agency?

A: Obviously, the first thing to look for is whether the agency offers the specific services you need. Some may offer nursing care, but not physical, occupational or speech therapy. Others may offer nursing care and therapy but no aides.

Equally important is the quality of services the agency provides. Licensing requirements for home health agencies vary from state to state. If your state licenses these agencies, check with the state health department to find out if the agency you are considering has a current, valid license. If your state does not license home-health agencies, find out if the agency is Medicare- or Medicaid-certified. Certification means not only that Medicare or Medicaid will cover services provided by the agency for their beneficiaries, it also means that the agency has met certain standards.

You should also determine if the facility is accredited. Two agencies—the Joint Commission on the Accreditation of Healthcare Organizations and the National League for Nursing—accredit home health agencies. Accreditation, which is voluntary, is like Medicare certification in that it indicates that the agency has met certain standards.

Q: **What exactly do home health aides and personal-care aides do?**

A: Home health aides, usually supervised by a nurse or therapist, can take vital signs, apply dressings, assist with exercises and walking, and help the survivor in activities of daily living, such as dressing, bathing, toileting and feeding. They may also provide light housekeeping services.

Personal-care aides, or home attendants, primarily assist the survivor in activities of daily living and help with housekeeping.

Q: I hadn't thought about housekeeping. I imagine it's virtually impossible for some stroke survivors and an extra burden on the caregiving family. Are there any other sources of housekeeping help out there?

A: Various housekeeping services—including cooking, shopping, doing laundry and cleaning—are offered by nonprofit agencies and volunteer programs sponsored by churches and other charitable organizations. Friends and extended family members can also be tapped to help out. And for those willing to pay, there are private housekeeping services.

Q: Where can I find out about these services?

A: Again, you can start by asking rehabilitation team members about the services available in your area. If your loved one is a senior citizen, your local area agency on aging may be another good starting point. These federally funded agencies, which are usually listed in the phone book's blue pages, track services and finance programs for older people who live at home. The blue pages may also help you locate other service agencies in your area—including Meals on Wheels, senior-citizen centers, and various other nonprofit and volunteer programs.

Q: Meals on Wheels is a meal service, right?

A: Yes. Meals on Wheels prepares and delivers meals for individuals who cannot prepare them themselves. This national nonprofit agency, which operates numerous local branches with the help of volunteers, may also help shut-ins with their grocery shopping. Area senior-citizen centers may also offer meals, although they usually require the recipient to come to the center to receive them.

Q: **Didn't you say there are also private companies that provide housekeeping services?**

A: There certainly are, although this is a more expensive route. A number of private housekeeping companies clean homes, prepare meals, shop and do laundry. Private laundry services also exist. Check your yellow pages to find the services available in your area. You might also consider hiring an independent housekeeper to provide whatever services you may need.

Q: **What about adult day care? What does it include?**

A: Adult day care is much like child day care—it provides the participant with needed supervision and stimulating activities in a safe, comfortable setting during specified hours—usually during the workweek. This service allows the caregiver to work, run errands or relax without worrying about leaving the stroke survivor unsupervised.

Like child day care, adult day care requires the adult to be taken to the day-care site. This means it may not be the best option for a stroke survivor who is either immobile or difficult to transport. It does, however, help alleviate the isolation common to stroke survivors. Adult day care not only provides the stroke survivor with supervision, it also provides him with opportunities to socialize with other adults.

Q: **Where can I find an adult day-care program?**

A: Practically unheard of a decade ago, adult day care is becoming more common as the need for it increases. Programs can be found in community centers and churches, as well as in independent facilities and even skilled nursing homes. To find a program or center in your area, consult the rehabilitation team or check the yellow pages of your phone book.

Q: **It sounds like adult day care gives the caregiver a needed break. What other kinds of respite care are there?**

A: Scheduled visits from a home health aide, personal-care aide, friend or family member can provide respite care for the primary caregiver, as can the survivor's temporary stay in a nursing home. Any situation that temporarily relieves the caregiver of the responsibility of caring for the stroke survivor can serve as a form of respite care.

Q: **Would you tell me more about checking services?**

A: Certainly. When a stroke survivor who lives alone is well enough to return home and wants to return to an independent lifestyle, his family and friends may respect his wishes but will probably have some concerns. Some of these concerns can be relieved by enlisting the services of one or more checking, or alerting, services. A service like this can monitor the survivor and alert family, friends or medical personnel to any possible problems.

The simplest of these services involves a simple daily phone call. Volunteers from a community organization or church, family members, friends or neighbors take turns calling the survivor once a day to see if everything is all right. In the case of a neighbor, a brief visit may replace the telephone call. This service, which costs nothing and can be set up by friends and family even in an area where it does not formally exist, also helps to keep the survivor in touch with others.

To provide survivors with a way to get help in an emergency situation, there are personal emergency-response systems—electronic signaling devices—that the survivor can either wear or carry. These devices connect to a response service, much like burglar alarms connect to security services or police departments. The survivor need only push a button or, if the device has an intercom function, push the button and state what's wrong, and the response service will alert the proper person and send help.

IRONING OUT THE DETAILS

Q: **Will all these home services be discussed when the discharge plan is prepared?**

A: Preparation of the discharge plan should include discussion not only about which services are necessary, but also about which services can and should be provided at home and which services can and should be provided on an outpatient basis. This discussion helps the rehabilitation team—including the survivor and family—determine the best way for the survivor to receive the services he needs. The discussion of services should also cover the costs of these services and whether or not they will be covered by the survivor's insurance policy.

Q: What do most insurance policies cover?

A: Most standard health-insurance policies cover a specified number of home health-care visits per year by participating home health agencies. The actual number of these visits varies according to individual policy. Covered visits generally include the services of nurses, dietitians and physical, speech and occupational therapists, as well as laboratory services and medical supplies. Housekeeping, companion and meal services are generally not covered.

Medicare and Medicaid also cover home health services as long as they are provided by a Medicare- or Medicaid-certified home health agency and are determined medically necessary by a doctor. Covered services include nursing care, physical, occupational and speech therapy, medical social services provided under the direction of a doctor, part-time or intermittent services of a home health aide, medical supplies (excluding drugs and biologicals) and durable medical equipment. Transportation and housekeeping services are not covered, although some Medicare supplemental policies do provide coverage for housekeeping, meal and companion services.

Q: Are there any specific questions a survivor or his family should ask before the actual move back home?

A: That depends on the status of the survivor and how well the rehabilitation team has prepared him and his family for the discharge. In general, however, he and the family will want to know:

　• if detailed instructions about medications, diet and therapy are included on the discharge plan;

　• if any prescribed medications produce side effects;

• how to determine if emergency medical care is needed;

• if there is anything specific the family needs to know about home care (e.g., how to administer medications, monitor blood pressure, deal with incontinence, assist in transferring the survivor from one place to another and so forth);

• what services, supplies and equipment will be needed, who will provide them and how they will be paid for;

• if there are specific exercises that should be done to preserve or regain physical abilities, and how often these exercises should be done;

• if there are any activities that should be avoided;

• which activities of daily living have been mastered, which are being worked on and how that work will continue;

• what, if any, adaptive equipment is available to make life at home simpler, and where to purchase that equipment;

• if there are any speech-therapy exercises that should be practiced at home and how often these exercises should be done;

• where family members can find counseling services after discharge and how they can contact any support groups in their area;

• who they can turn to for answers to questions that arise after the survivor has returned home.

Q: You mentioned support groups. What types are available?

A: A number of support groups are available for stroke survivors and their families. Many areas have regional **stroke clubs**, which enable stroke survivors and their families to meet each other, share their experiences and offer advice and support. Members of the rehabilitation team may be able to put you in touch with a local club, or you may find a local club listed in the blue pages of your phone book. Some hospitals and rehabilitation centers offer their own support groups for their patients. And several national organizations offer assistance in establishing stroke support groups where none exist. Stroke survivors may also participate in support groups designed for people with specific disabilities, such as paralysis and aphasia. And support groups are also available for caregivers and family members of stroke survivors. For more information about support groups, see the section "Informational and Mutual-Aid Groups."

Q: How long will the need for such support groups continue?

A: That depends on the individual stroke survivor and his family. Returning home is a major step forward in the rehabilitation process, but it is not the end. The stroke survivor and his family still have a long road ahead of them and may need support for months, or even years, to come.

8 WHAT FAMILIES SHOULD KNOW

Q: It seems as though the lives of family members can be affected by stroke almost as much as the lives of stroke survivors. Am I right?

A: Yes. Stroke can be considered a family illness— it affects every member in some way. It prompts strong emotional reactions, affects behavior, lifestyle and relationships, and alters family roles. Family members not only must come to grips with the physical, cognitive and emotional changes in their loved one—an emotionally draining experience in itself—they must also serve as a major source of emotional, social and practical support.

Q: So it's normal for family members to feel overwhelmed?

A: It certainly is. Feelings of frustration, anger, insecurity, self-pity, uncertainty, impatience, guilt, resentfulness, loneliness, isolation and sadness are also normal.

After the initial shock and worry wear off, family members may feel sorry for themselves or angry at their situation. As their loved one progresses through therapy and her various impairments and changes are revealed, they may grieve for the loss of their loved one as she used to be. They may be frustrated by the slowness of the rehabilitation process or their own inability to change things. Feelings of inadequacy may also arise when they assume caregiving roles. They may feel insecure about their own abilities and uncertain about the future. They may find themselves so wrapped up in caring for their loved one that they cut themselves off from their normal social life and end up feeling lonely and isolated. And when they do take some time for themselves or reflect on their negative feelings, they may feel guilty. This is all perfectly normal. After all, their lives and the life of their loved one have changed suddenly in a manner over which they've had little or no control and for which they've had little or no preparation.

Q: **What aspect of stroke is hardest for family members to deal with?**

A: That depends on the family, its situation and the situation of the stroke survivor. For some it's dealing with personality, role or lifestyle changes; for others, it's dealing with caregiving responsibilities.

DEALING WITH CHANGES

Q: **Refresh my memory. What kind of personality changes might stroke survivors undergo?**

A: Stroke survivors may experience a decrease in motivation or self-control; they may become frustrated, impatient or irritable; or they may behave rashly or impulsively or slowly and compulsively. They may suddenly become overtalkative or socially withdrawn. They may deny their limitations or become totally apathetic. They may behave in socially inappropriate ways, demonstrating selfishness, insensitivity and tactlessness or throwing temper tantrums. And they may be unable to control their emotions.

Q: How can family members deal with these changes?

A: Primarily by learning to accept them. Although the family members naturally want their loved ones to return to the way they were, they must accept them the way they are. Family members need to realize that the changes are the result of brain injury; they are not deliberate attempts to "act out." They also need to realize that many stroke survivors are not aware of these personality changes: Simply telling survivors to act normally has little or no effect.

Family members can, however, establish behavioral limits. They can set rules and enforce those rules. While they should not talk down to a stroke survivor or treat him like a child, they should indicate what type of behavior will and will not be tolerated and follow through on those rules.

Q: How should the family deal with the stroke survivor's uncontrollable emotional outbursts?

A: Often the best way to deal with emotional lability is to ignore it. Remember, however, that other people who know the survivor may not be aware of this somewhat disturbing effect. Family members may need to explain emotional lability and other behavioral and personality changes to friends and others who are taken aback by this behavior.

Q: What about other aspects of the survivor's emotional state? Is there anything family members should do?

A: Family members need to be aware of their loved one's emotional state and be able to recognize the signs of depression (see Chapter 6), so they can get help, if needed. But even a survivor who is not depressed can benefit from his family's efforts to maintain his self-esteem and reduce his isolation. The family needs to make the survivor feel at home and let him control as much of his life as he can, so he can be as independent as possible. They can assign him small tasks to make him feel needed, and they can encourage friends and other family members to visit, to stimulate social interaction.

Family members also need to be aware of their own emotional states. They should realize that they, too, are susceptible to depression and isolation. They should make efforts to socialize and express their emotions. And they should feel free to seek counseling, if needed.

Q: How can families deal with the changes in family roles and lifestyles?

A: Again, primarily by learning to accept them. This can be quite difficult for both the family and stroke survivor, and it may take time. It is difficult for a spouse to change from partner to caregiver; it is difficult for an adult son or daughter to suddenly be responsible for caring for a parent; and it is difficult for a parent to accept care from a child.

Likewise, it is difficult for the family breadwinner to accept being unable to work, or a nonworking spouse to suddenly enter the workforce. Giving up or assuming new household roles, too, can be difficult. The family's former financial manager, for example, may feel inadequate and out of control when the books are transferred to another family member. And that family member may be over-whelmed by the financial responsibilities.

All these changes require adjustment; some require education and training, and all may be made a little easier with the help of counseling and support groups—for all involved. Education, training and counseling also make it easier for family members to assume caregiving responsibilities.

DEALING WITH CAREGIVING RESPONSIBILITIES

Q: **What caregiving responsibilities do family members assume?**

A: That depends on the stroke survivor's needs and the family members' abilities. Most family members offer needed emotional support and encouragement without thinking. After all, the stroke survivor is someone they love and care about. Depending on the needs of that survivor, however, family members may also address physical needs, helping with therapy, walking, transferring, eating, dressing, bathing and toileting. Generally, however, they need some type of training before they can assume these responsibilities.

Q: **Where do family members get this training?**

A: Primarily from the rehabilitation team. Family members may, for example, observe physical, occupational and speech-therapy sessions, asking numerous questions of the therapists. They may then ask the

therapist how they can assist their loved one with therapy.
The therapists are usually happy to comply, giving the
family instructions in how to help their loved one with
the exercises that are so important to his recovery. They
may learn from the therapists and the nursing staff how to
help their loved one stand up, balance and sit down, or
how to transfer from one resting spot to another. Or they
may ask the occupational therapist how they can best
help their loved one dress herself or eat. In general, they
learn from watching the experts and asking the experts
for instructions.

Q: What other responsibilities do caregiving family members assume?

A: If the stroke has caused cognitive or perceptual problems that affect the survivor's judgment,
family caregivers may need to provide constant super-
vision to prevent their loved one from injuring herself.
They may also take responsibility for reducing their loved
one's risk of suffering another stroke, perhaps by watching
her diet or making sure she takes prescribed medications.

Q: It sounds like caregiving can be a full-time occupation! Is there any relief for the family members?

A: There is. As we discussed in Chapter 7, numerous services provide assistance to a family who is caring
for its loved one at home. Home health aides, personal-
care aides, housekeeping services, laundry services and
meal services can all lessen the responsibilities.

In addition, the primary caregiver should feel free to
share responsibilities with other members of the family
and friends. Many caregivers make the mistake of trying

to do everything themselves. This takes a tremendous toll on their health and well-being, in that caregiving can be fatiguing. It doesn't end when the clock strikes five, and it requires both physical and emotional stamina. Caregivers need a break.

Q: Are you talking about respite care?

A: Yes. Respite care—for several weeks or several hours—is essential to caregivers, who are almost as likely to become isolated and lonely as stroke survivors. Caregivers need to take some time for themselves—to exercise, relax, reduce stress and socialize. This is important for their health and well-being, and ultimately, the health and well-being of their loved one.

Q: You've mentioned counseling and support groups several times. What type of services are available for families and caregivers?

A: In addition to individual or group counseling from a psychologist or psychiatrist, family members may also benefit from family therapy or from participation in one or more support groups. Most stroke clubs welcome family members, and some hospitals and rehabilitation centers set up support groups just for family members and caregivers. In addition, there are support groups specifically designed for adult children of aging parents and for caregivers. To find a support group, check with the members of the rehabilitation team, consult the blue pages of your telephone directory or see the section "Informational and Mutual-Aid Groups."

Q: To sum up, do you have any general advice to help family members deal with their loved one's stroke and recovery?

A: Certainly.

• Take an active role in your loved one's medical care and rehabilitation.

• Learn as much as you can about stroke.

• Divide and share responsibilities.

• Learn what community services are available and take advantage of them.

• Realize that it takes time to adjust to altered personalities and changed roles.

• Don't be afraid to express your feelings.

• Be aware of your own needs, and don't hesitate to satisfy them.

• Take advantage of counseling, support groups and offers of help from friends.

INFORMATIONAL
AND
MUTUAL-AID GROUPS

American Heart Association
Stroke Connection
7272 Greenville Ave.
Dallas, TX 75231
800-553-6321

> *Provides information and referrals; maintains support-group information; offers peer counseling to stroke survivors and caregivers; publishes* Stroke Connection *magazine.*

American Occupational Therapy Association
4720 Montgomery Ln.
P.O. Box 31220
Bethesda, MD 20824-1220
301-652-2682

> *National professional organization for occupational therapists. Provides state contact information for people seeking occupational therapists.*

American Speech-Language-Hearing Association
10801 Rockville Pike
Rockville, MD 20852
301-897-5700
800-638-8255

> *Professional organization for speech-language pathologists. Provides information on speech, language and hearing problems and referrals to qualified speech-language pathologists.*

Children of Aging Parents
1609 Woodbourne Rd., Suite 302A
Levittown, PA 19057-1511
215-945-6900

> *Provides information and referrals to caregivers of the elderly; assists in starting support groups; publishes bimonthly newsletter. Annual family membership, $20.*

Commission on the Accreditation of Rehabilitation Facilities
101 N. Wilmot Rd., Suite 500
Tucson, AZ 85711
602-748-1212

> *Accredits rehabilitation centers.*

Elder Care Locator
800-677-1118

> *A public service of the U.S. Department of Health and Human Services' Administration on Aging. Helps people locate local services and resources for senior citizens.*

Joint Commission on Accreditation of Healthcare Organizations
1 Renaissance Blvd.
Oakbrook Terrace, IL 60181
708-916-5600

> *Accredits rehabilitation centers and home health agencies.*

Medical Rehabilitation Education Foundation
1910 Association Dr.
Reston, VA 22091
800-GET REHAB (438-7342)

> *Provides information on and referrals to medical rehabilitation facilities.*

National Aphasia Association
P.O. Box 1887
Murray Hill Station
New York, NY 10156-0611
800-922-4622

Provides information about aphasia and referrals to local support groups; provides information on starting support groups; publishes biannual newsletter.

National Easter Seal Society
230 W. Monroe, Suite 1800
Chicago, IL 60606
312-726-6200
800-221-6827

Designed to help people with disabilities achieve independence; provides information on local Easter Seal societies and the programs and services they offer. Many Easter Seal societies provide services to stroke patients and have stroke clubs.

National Family Caregivers Association
9621 E. Bexhill Dr.
Kensington, MD 20895-3104
301-942-6430
800-896-3650

Provides information, education and support to family caregivers; operates an information clearinghouse; provides educational materials and speakers; advocates respite care; publishes quarterly newsletter. Membership, $15.

NIDCD Clearinghouse
1 Communications Ave.
Bethesda, MD 20892-3456
800-241-1044

Clearinghouse for the National Institute on Deafness and Other Communication Disorders; offers publications on aphasia; can provide other information on aphasia via a computer database.

National Institute of Neurological Disorders and Stroke
Neurological Institute
P.O. Box 5801
Bethesda, MD 20824
800-352-9424

> Provides information on a wide range of neurological diseases, including stroke. Offers publications.

National League for Nursing
350 Hudson St.
New York, NY 10014
212-989-9393

> Accredits home health agencies.

National Meals on Wheels Foundation
2675 44th St. S.W., Suite 305
Grand Rapids, MI 49509
800-999-6262
616-531-9909

> Provides information on Meals on Wheels program; offers referrals to local chapters.

National Rehabilitation Information Center
8455 Colesville Rd., Suite 935
Silver Spring, MD 20910
800-346-2742
301-588-9284

> Provides information on disabilities, rehabilitation and related issues; publishes a stroke resource guide.

National Stroke Association
8480 E. Orchard Rd., Suite 1000
Englewood, CO 80111-5015
303-771-1700
800-STROKE (787-6537)

> *Provides information on strokes; offers counseling and assistance; offers referrals to organizations establishing stroke programs and support groups; provides materials on stroke prevention, treatment and care; sells publications and videos; publishes the* Journal of Stroke and Cerebrovascular Disease; *and the* Be Stroke Smart *newsletter. Individual memberships ($20) include a newsletter subscription and a discount on publications.*

Stroke Clubs International
805 Twelfth St.
Galveston, TX 77550
409-762-1022

> *Refers individuals to information sources and local stroke support groups.*

Visiting Nurse Associations of America
3801 E. Florida Ave., Suite 900
Denver, CO 80210
800-426-2547
303-753-0218

> *Provides referrals to local Visiting Nurse Associations around the country.*

Well Spouse Foundation
610 Lexington Ave., Suite 814
New York, NY 10022
212-644-1241
800-838-0879

> *Offers support to spouses and partners of chronically ill or disabled individuals; provides referrals to existing local support groups; aids in establishing local support groups; publishes bimonthly newsletter.*

SOURCES FOR ADAPTIVE CLOTHING AND EQUIPMENT

CLEO, Inc.
70 S. Buckhout St.
Irvington, NY 10533
800-321-0595

Enrichments
P.O. Box 471
Western Springs, IL 60558
800-323-5547

Maddak, Inc.
Pequannock, NJ 07440-1993
800-443-4926

Patient's Personal Needs, Inc.
275 Centre St.
Holbrook, MA 02343
800-289-4776

Wardrobe Wagon, Inc.
555 Valley Rd.
West Orange, NJ 07052
800-992-2737

Glossary

Activities of daily living: Normal everyday actions, such as eating, drinking, dressing and grooming.

Agnosia: Inability to recognize familiar objects or to associate an object with its use.

Anemia: A condition in which the blood is deficient in red blood cells, in hemoglobin or in total volume; a possible consequence of sickle-cell disease.

Aneurysm: A weak spot in the wall of a blood vessel. An aneurysm can rupture and cause bleeding.

Angiogram: An x-ray picture of a blood vessel.

Angiography: An imaging procedure that enables blood vessels to be seen on film after the vessels have been filled with a contrast medium; dye is injected into the blood, then x-rays are taken.

Anomia: The inability to recall the names of familiar objects.

Anticoagulant: A drug that helps prevent or delay blood clots; a *blood thinner.*

Aphasia: Inability to express oneself in language or to understand the language of others.

Apoplexy: Old term for stroke.

Apraxia: Inability to voluntarily perform skilled movements.

Arrhythmia: An abnormal heart rhythm.

Arteriogram: An angiogram of an artery.

Aspiration pneumonia: An inflammation of the lungs and bronchial tubes caused by taking foreign material into the lungs; often a complication of stroke.

Ataxia: Impaired movement; lack of coordination, unsteady gait and poor balance.

Atherosclerosis: Condition in which the inner layers of the artery walls become thick and irregular due to deposits of fat, cholesterol and other substances.

Atrial fibrillation: A type of irregular heartbeat in which the upper chambers of the heart (atria) beat irregularly and very rapidly; a risk factor for stroke.

Balloon angioplasty: A procedure for treating a narrowing or blockage of a blood vessel; a catheter with a deflated balloon on its tip is passed into the narrowed artery segment, the balloon is inflated and the narrowed segment gets widened.

Barium swallow: X-ray pictures of the esophagus, stomach and duodenum taken after a person swallows barium sulfate; used to locate problems that might be causing swallowing and digestive problems.

Basilar artery: Artery at the base of the skull that supplies blood to some parts of the brain.

Beginning spasticity: Stage in which muscle tone begins to return to a paralyzed area.

B-mode imaging: A form of ultrasound that provides three-dimensional images.

Brain stem: Part of the brain that connects it to the spine; controls motor, sense and reflex functions.

Bruit: An abnormal sound.

Cardiologist: A doctor who specializes in treating heart problems.

Carotid arteries: Arteries that bring blood from the heart to the brain via the neck.

Carotid endarterectomy: Surgical removal of plaque deposits or blood clots in the carotid artery.

Cerebellum: Part of the brain that controls movement coordination.

Cerebral embolism: Clot or other material that originates somewhere in the body, travels through the bloodstream, and lodges in and blocks an artery supplying the brain.

Cerebral hemorrhage: Bleeding within the brain caused by the leakage or rupture of a blood vessel or by a head injury.

Cerebral infarction: Another term for **ischemic stroke**.

Cerebral thrombosis: Formation of a clot in an artery supplying the brain with blood.

Cerebrovascular accident (CVA): See **Stroke**.

Cerebrum: The largest, uppermost section of the brain; divided into two hemispheres—left and right.

Checking services: Any of a number of services designed to check in on a stroke survivor who lives alone.

Cholesterol: A fatlike substance found in animal tissue and produced by the human body. Cholesterol helps the body absorb and move fatty acids and manufacture hormones.

Computerized axial tomography (CAT): A computer-enhanced series of cross-sectional x-ray images of selected parts of the body. Also called *computerized tomography (CT).*

Computerized tomography (CT): See **Computerized axial tomography (CAT).**

Contractures: Shortening or tightening of tissue around a joint that prevents the joint and surrounding muscles from moving.

Custodial care: Room, board and personal care.

Cytoprotective: Protecting cells; cytoprotective drugs protect cells from damage.

Decubitus ulcer: Bedsore, pressure ulcer; a swollen sore or ulcer of the skin over a bony part of the body resulting from prolonged pressure; a complication of stroke.

Diastolic: The measurement of blood pressure when the heart is in its resting or relaxation phase; the lower number in a blood-pressure reading.

Discharge plan: Written plan that outlines the treatment and care a stroke patient should receive after discharge from the hospital or rehabilitation center.

Diuretics: Drugs that promote urination, thus speeding the elimination of sodium and water; often used to control blood pressure.

Doppler scanning: Ultrasound technique that monitors the behavior of something that moves, such as blood.

Dysarthria: Imperfect speech articulation due to muscular-control problems caused by damage to the brain or nervous system.

Dysmetria: Perceptual impairment that prevents a person from accurately estimating distances linked to muscle movements.

Dysphagia: Difficulty swallowing.

Edema: The swelling of body tissue.

Electrocardiogram (EKG): A graphic record of electrical impulses produced by the heart.

Electroencephalogram (EEG): Diagnostic test in which electrodes are put on the scalp to pick up electrical impulses transmitted and received by the brain cells.

Embolism: Blockage of a blood vessel by a clot or other foreign material carried by the bloodstream from one part of the body to another; a cause of stroke.

Embolus: A solid particle, usually a fragment of clotted blood or a fatty deposit, carried along in the bloodstream.

Evacuation: Surgical procedure in which a substance is drained, removed or evacuated from a cavity, space or organ of the body.

Evoked response: Tests that measure how the brain responds to sensory stimuli; a doctor stimulates the senses and monitors the patient's response.

Expressive aphasia: An inability to say or write known words—in other words, an inability to express oneself—caused by brain damage.

Fibrinogen: A protein in the blood-clotting process.

Flaccidity: Absence of muscle tone and reflexive and voluntary movement.

Full spasticity: Stage of paralysis in which muscles are unusually tense and resistant to stretching.

Geriatrician: Doctor who specializes in dealing with diseases of the elderly and the problems associated with aging.

Global aphasia: The inability to speak, write or understand written or verbal speech, caused by damage to the brain.

Glutamate cascade: Chemical chain reaction in the brain, triggered by ischemic brain cells, that results in the death of or damage to surrounding brain cells.

Hematoma: A collection of blood that has escaped from the vessels and has become trapped in the tissues of the skin or in an organ.

Hemianesthesia: Loss of sensation in one half of the body.

Hemianopia: Damage to optic nerve resulting in blindness in half of each eye.

Hemiparesis: Weakness on one side of body.

Hemiplegia: Paralysis on one side of body.

Hemorrhagic stroke: Cerebrovascular accident caused by the rupture or leakage of blood vessels in or on the brain.

Heparin: Anticoagulant drug that reduces the tendency of the blood to clot; a *blood thinner.*

Home health agency: An organization that provides health care in the home.

Home health aide: A worker who assists in providing health- and personal-care services to a patient living at home.

Hypertension: A chronic increase in blood pressure above its normal range; generally, systolic readings greater than 140 and/or diastolic readings greater than 90 over a period of time.

Hypoperfusion: Decreased blood flow to an organ.

Hypotension: Low blood pressure.

Infarct: Area of tissue that is dead or dying, having been deprived of blood.

Intermediate-care facility: Nursing home that provides health care and services to people who do not require the care and services of a hospital or skilled nursing facility.

Ischemia: A localized deficiency of blood flow, usually due to obstruction of a blood vessel.

Ischemic stroke: Cerebrovascular accident caused by insufficient blood flow to the brain.

Jargon aphasia: Communication disorder in which a person will repeat one or more words without context.

Lability: Instability.

Left ventricular hypertrophy (LVH): Condition in which the heart's left ventricle is enlarged; a risk factor for stroke.

Lumbar puncture: A sampling of cerebrospinal fluid removed from the spinal canal by means of a long needle; used to diagnose diseases of and injuries to the brain and spinal cord, including stroke.

Magnetic resonance angiography: Test that uses magnetic fields and radio waves to create images of blood vessels.

Magnetic resonance imaging (MRI): A diagnostic technique that provides high-quality cross-sectional images of organs and structures in the body using a magnetic field (instead of radiation).

Management plan: See **Discharge plan**.

Neglect: Perceptual impairment resulting in lack of awareness of one side of the body.

Neurologist: Doctor who specializes in the brain and nervous system.

Neurosurgeon: Surgeon who specializes in the nervous system (brain, spinal cord and nerves).

Neurotransmitter: A chemical that assists in sending signals among nerve cells.

Nimodipine: A calcium channel blocking drug.

Nuclear brain scan: Imaging test that uses radioactive material to produce a picture of the brain.

Occlusion: Blockage of any passage, canal, vessel or opening of the body.

Occupational therapist: An allied health professional who helps disabled people regain fulfilling daily occupations of leisure and work.

Ocular plethysmography: Test that measures blood pressure in the eyes.

Ophthalmodynamometry: Test to determine the blood pressure in the eye's retinal artery.

Paraphasia: Partial aphasia in which a person uses the wrong words or sounds.

Paresthesia: Numbness or tingling feeling.

Partially reversible ischemic neurological deficit (PRIND): A minor stroke in which symptoms last longer than three days but produce only minor dysfunction.

Penumbra: Area surrounding an infarct, which can itself become injured.

Personal-care aide: Worker who provides services that help a person meet the demands of daily living.

Phonoangiography: The recording and analysis of arterial bruits to estimate the extent of stenosis.

Physiatrist: Doctor who specializes in physical medicine.

Physical therapist: An allied health professional, trained and licensed in physical therapy, who helps physically disabled individuals regain functional movement, heal and adapt to their disabilities.

Plaque: A deposit of fatty (and other) substances in the inner lining of the artery wall characteristic of atherosclerosis.

Platelet inhibitors: Drugs that prevent platelets from collecting; *blood thinners.*

Polycythemia: Condition in which there is an increased number of red blood cells in blood.

Positron emission tomography (PET): A technique for making computer-generated images of the brain or other body organs by means of radioactive isotopes injected into the body; used to locate abnormal tissue.

Pulmonary embolism: An embolism that lodges in the pulmonary artery or in another vessel in a lung.

Radioactive isotopes: Unstable forms of an element, which give off radiation as the nuclei of their atoms decay.

Radionuclide angiography: Technique that uses radioactive isotopes to create images of inner parts of the body.

Range of motion (ROM): The range through which a joint can be extended and flexed.

Receptive aphasia: Form of aphasia in which a person cannot understand spoken or written language.

Recreational therapist: Allied health professional who uses games and other activities to increase social activity as part of rehabilitation.

Rehabilitation: Restoring an individual to maximum physical, mental, social, spiritual and vocational potential.

Rehabilitation center: A facility that provides medical, health-related, social and/or vocational services to disabled people to help them attain their maximum functional capacity.

Residential care home: A facility, such as a nursing home, that provides custodial care for people who are unable to live by themselves.

Respite care: Temporary care for a person whose care or supervision is normally provided by family members at home; respite care gives family members temporary relief from caregiving demands.

Reversible ischemic neurological deficit (RIND): Minor stroke whose symptoms last more than one day but leave only minor deficits.

Sickle-cell disease: Inherited condition in which red blood cells have an abnormal, crescent shape.

Skilled nursing facility: A nursing home that provides skilled nursing care and related services for seriously ill patients who require inpatient medical or nursing care similar to that received in a hospital.

Spasticity: Increase in normal tension of a muscle, resulting in a continuous resistance to stretching.

Speech-language pathologist: An allied health professional who measures and evaluates language and speech-production abilities and clinically treats individuals with speech and language disorders.

Speech therapist: See **Speech-language pathologist**.

Spinal tap: See **Lumbar puncture**.

Stenosis: The narrowing or constriction of an opening, such as a blood vessel.

Stroke: Sudden loss of function of part of the brain due to an interference in blood supply.

Stroke Belt: Area of Southeastern United States where more strokes occur: States include Indiana, Kentucky, Virginia, Arkansas, Tennessee, North Carolina, South Carolina, Georgia, Alabama, Mississippi and Louisiana.

Stroke clubs: Support groups for stroke survivors and their families.

Subarachnoid hemorrhage: Bleeding between the arachnoid membrane and the surface of the brain; often caused by a ruptured aneurysm.

Subluxation: Dislocation, usually of the shoulder joint.

Systolic: The measurement of blood pressure when the left ventricle contracts and the blood's force against the vessel walls is at its greatest strength; the higher number in a blood-pressure reading.

Thrombolytic: Clot-dissolving.

Thrombosis: Formation, development or presence of a blood clot in a blood vessel; can cause stroke.

Thrombus: A blood clot.

Ticlopidine: A platelet inhibitor used to prevent and treat stroke.

Tissue plasminogen activator (tPA): A genetically engineered enzyme that dissolves blood clots.

Transcranial Doppler: Noninvasive, ultrasound test that produces images of blood flow in the brain.

Transfer: A move from one sitting or resting position to another.

Transient ischemic attack (TIA): A temporary strokelike event that lasts less than 24 hours and is caused by a temporarily blocked blood vessel.

Ultrasound: A picture of organs and structures inside the body made with high-frequency sound waves.

Urologist: Doctor who specializes in diagnosing and treating diseases of the urinary system.

Vasospasm: A sudden, short-term spasm of a blood vessel; a complication of subarachnoid hemorrhage.

Ventriculostomy: Surgical drainage of spinal fluid and blood from the brain's ventricles.

Verbal apraxia: Communication disorder in which the brain has difficulty sending messages regarding speech movement to the speech muscles.

Vertebral arteries: Arteries that carry blood to the deep neck muscles, spine and parts of the brain.

Warfarin: An anticoagulant drug used in stroke prevention and treatment.

SUGGESTED READING

Ahn, Jung, M.D., and Gary Ferguson. *Recovery From a Stroke: A Doctor's Guide for Patients and Their Loved Ones.* New York: Harper Paperbacks, 1992.

Ancowitz, Arthur, M.D. *The Stroke Book: One-on-One Advice About Stroke Prevention, Management and Rehabilitation.* New York: William Morrow and Company, Inc., 1993.

Caplan, Louis R., M.D., Mark L. Dyken, M.D., and J. Donald Easton, M.D. *The American Heart Association Family Guide to Stroke Treatment, Recovery and Prevention.* New York: Times Books, 1994.

Caplan, Louis R., M.D., and Robert W. Stein, M.D. *Stroke: A Clinical Approach.* Stoneham, Mass.: Butterworth Publishing, 1986.

Donnan, Geoffrey, M.D., and Carol Burton. *After a Stroke: A Support Book for Patients, Caregivers, Families and Friends.* Berkeley, Calif.: North Atlantic Books, 1990.

Foley, Conn, M.D., and H.F. Pizer, PA-C. *The Stroke Fact Book: Everything You Want and Need to Know About Stroke—From Prevention to Rehabilitation.* Golden Valley, Minn.: Courage Press, 1990.

Frye-Pierson, Janice, R.N., B.S.N., CNRN, and James F. Toole, M.D. *Stroke: A Guide for Patient and Family.* New York: Raven Press, 1987.

Josephs, Arthur. *The Invaluable Guide to Life After Stroke: An Owner's Manual.* Long Beach, Calif.: Amadeus Press, 1992.

National Stroke Association. *The Road Ahead: A Stroke Recovery Guide.* Englewood, Col.: National Stroke Association, 1988.

Rose, F. Clifford, and Rudy Capildeo. *Stroke: The Facts.* New York: Oxford University Press, 1981.

Shimberg, Elaine Fantle. *Strokes: What Families Should Know.* New York: Ballantine Books, 1990.

Shirk, Evelyn Urban. *After the Stroke: Coping With America's Third Leading Cause of Death.* Buffalo, N.Y.: Prometheus Books, 1991.

Singleton, Lafayette, M.D., and Kirk Johnson. *The Black Health Library Guide to Stroke.* New York: Henry Holt and Co., 1993.

INDEX

A

ACE inhibitors, stroke recurrence and, 100
Acetaminophen, fever in ischemic stroke and, 87
Activities of daily living
defined, 27, 165
home care and, 141, 147
Adaptive clothing, sources, 163
Adaptive equipment
home care, 147
sources, 163
Adult day care, 143-144
Age
hypertension and, 47
stroke and, 35-37
Agnosia, defined, 21, 165
Alcohol, effects, 65-66
Anemia
defined, 165
in sickle-cell disease, 38
Aneurysm, defined, 30, 165
Angiogram, defined, 80, 165
Angiography. *See also* Magnetic resonance angiography
conventional vs. magnetic resonance, 79-80
defined, 79, 165

Angioplasty. *See also* Balloon angioplasty
ischemic stroke and, 91
Anomia, defined, 18, 165
Antibiotics, infection and, 100
Anticoagulants
atrial fibrillation and, 56-57
blocked carotid arteries and, 54
defined, 165
general uses, 57
ischemic stroke and, 88-89
pulmonary embolism and, 100
transient ischemic attack (TIA) and, 165
Anticonvulsants, seizures and, 100
Antidepressants, depression and, 100, 127
Antihypertensives
blocked carotid arteries and, 54
types, 48
Apathy, 23
Aphasia. *See also* Expressive aphasia; Global aphasia; Jargon aphasia; Receptive aphasia
defined, 18, 165
Apoplexy, defined, 25, 166
Arm function, restoration, 117
Arm troughs, 115